Atherosclerosis, Arteriosclerosis and Arteriolosclerosis

Edited by Luigi Gianturco

Published in London, United Kingdom

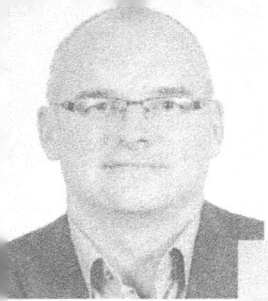
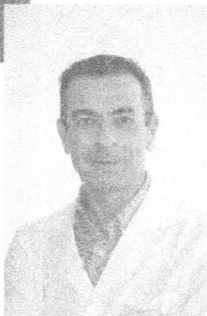
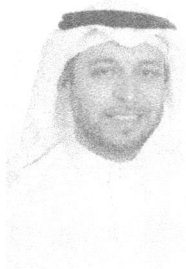
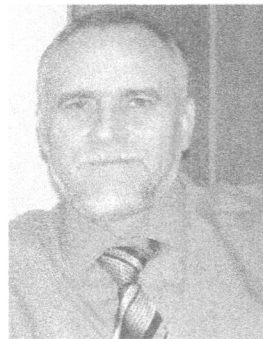
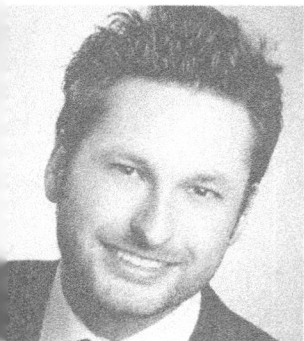
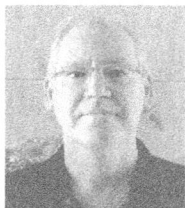
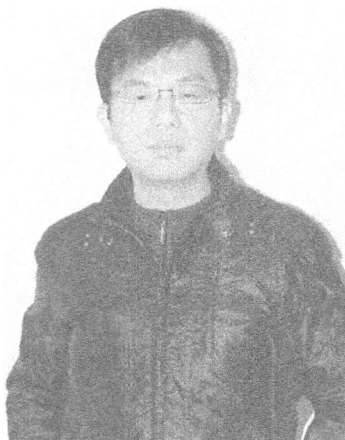

IntechOpen

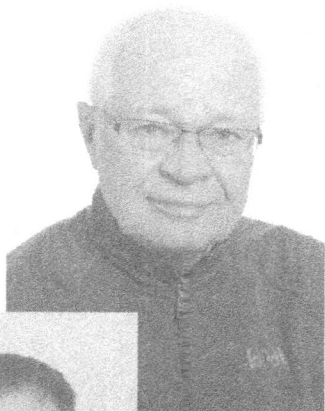
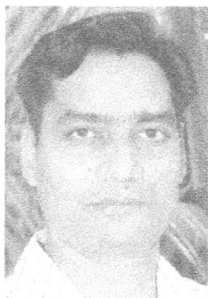
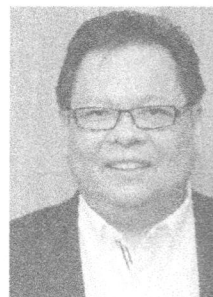
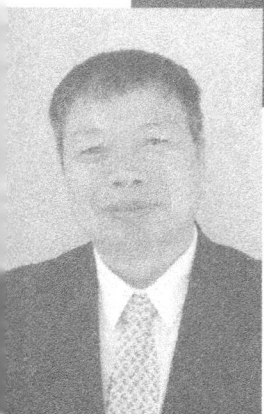
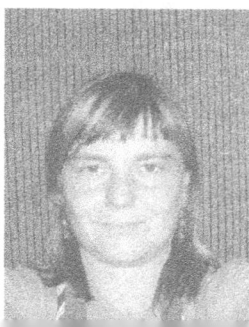
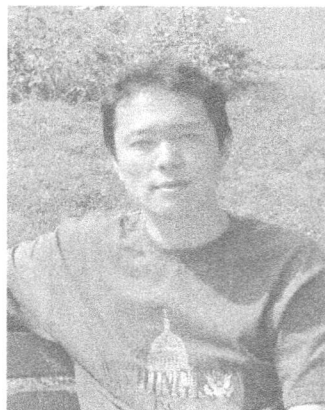

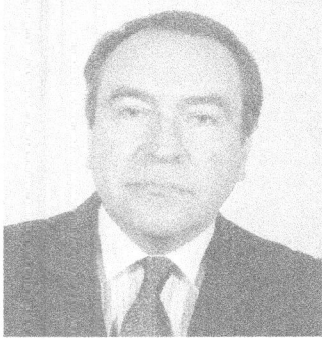

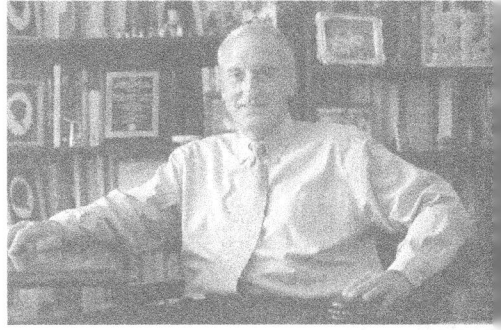

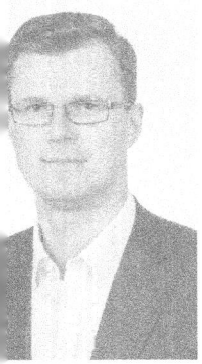

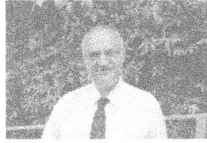

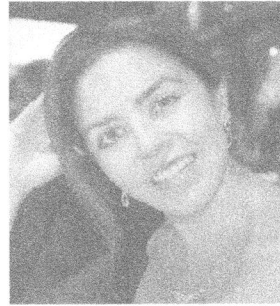

Supporting open minds since 2005

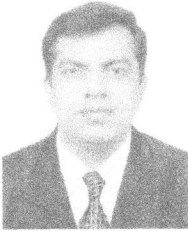

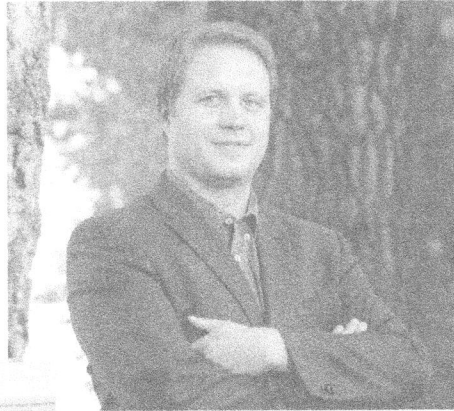

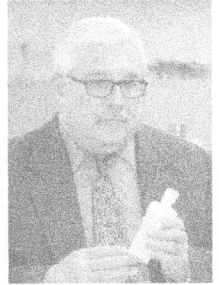

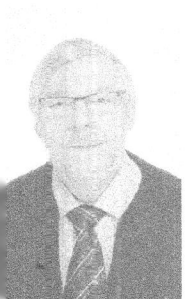

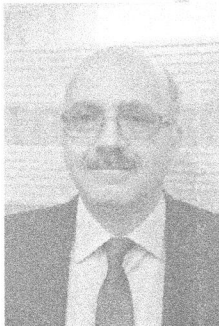

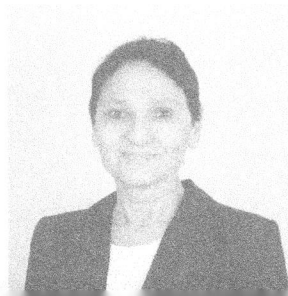

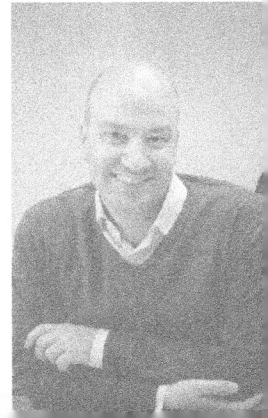

Atherosclerosis, Arteriosclerosis and Arteriolosclerosis
http://dx.doi.org/10.5772/intechopen.83058
Edited by Luigi Gianturco

Contributors
Lena Lavie, Michal Tomcik, Sabina Oreska, Minerva Irene Hernández Rejón, Manuel Alexis Vargas Robles,
Oladimeji Adebayo, Abiodun Moshood Adeoye, Nishtha Sareen, Abhishek Ojha, Luigi Gianturco

Notice
Statements and opinions expressed in the chapters are these of the individual contributors and not
necessarily those of the editors or publisher. No responsibility is accepted for the accuracy of
information contained in the published chapters. The publisher assumes no responsibility for any
damage or injury to persons or property arising out of the use of any materials, instructions, methods
or ideas contained in the book.

First published in London, United Kingdom, 2020 by IntechOpen
IntechOpen is the global imprint of INTECHOPEN LIMITED, registered in England and Wales,
registration number: 11086078, 7th floor, 10 Lower Thames Street, London,
EC3R 6AF, United Kingdom
Printed in Croatia

British Library Cataloguing-in-Publication Data
A catalogue record for this book is available from the British Library

Additional hard and PDF copies can be obtained from orders@intechopen.com

Atherosclerosis, Arteriosclerosis and Arteriolosclerosis
Edited by Luigi Gianturco
p. cm.
Print ISBN 978-1-83880-303-2
Online ISBN 978-1-83880-304-9
eBook (PDF) ISBN 978-1-83880-524-1

We are IntechOpen,
the world's leading publisher of
Open Access books

Built by scientists, for scientists

4,800+
Open access books available

122,000+
International authors and editors

135M+
Downloads

Our authors are among the

151
Countries delivered to

Top 1%
most cited scientists

12.2%
Contributors from top 500 universities

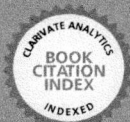

Interested in publishing with us?
Contact book.department@intechopen.com

Numbers displayed above are based on latest data collected.
For more information visit www.intechopen.com

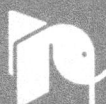

Meet the editor

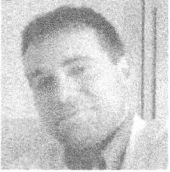

Luigi Gianturco, MD, MSc, obtained his MD cum laude in Medicine and Surgery with a specialty in Cardiology from Sapienza University of Rome in July 2003 and November 2007, respectively. He also obtained an MSc in Clinical Echocardiography from the University of Milan in 2009. Currently, Dr. Gianturco works in the Cardio Rehab Unit of Passirana-Rho Hospital. Previously, he was Vice-Chief of the Cardiology Unit at Galeazzi Orthopedic Institute, Milan, and Assistant Manager of inside clinical risk management and overall health direction unit. He has made several oral presentations at national and international conventions and published works in national and international journals. He has also served as an investigator in some important national and international studies. He has been a member of the Italian Soccer Referees' Medical Committee since 2013. Dr. Gianturco has a great passion for reading and writing, and runs a personal blog at www.luigigianturco.com.

Contents

Preface

Despite a reduction in deaths over the last two decades, atherosclerosis (ATS) is still a major concern worldwide. Decreased mortality can be attributed to anti-smoking laws, especially in Western countries, as it is well established that smoking may accelerate ATS injury. Unfortunately, ATS morbidity and mortality are still quite high. Nowadays, the major cardiovascular risk (CVR) factors contributing to ATS are "metabolic" and include such conditions as dyslipidemia, diabetes, and metabolic syndrome. As such, we understand how global cardiovascular disease (CVD) determines about 30% of world deaths, and ATS is definitely a pivotal contributor to CVD. Although there is much in the literature about ATS, the discussions seem to cover most of the same topics. This book, however, covers not only those topics but also less debated subjects.

For example, you are going to read about the link between CVD and obstructive sleep apneas (the so-called OSAs). Last evidences have linked OSAs to multiple CV disorders including diabetes and coronary artery disease (CAD). Very often, the determinants of ATS progression and OSAs are common and thus it is pivotal to address the linkage between them.

In this volume, you will also find a discussion about the consolidated and close relationship of rheumatology and CV risk. In particular, several contributing authors have been studying how and/or how much systemic rheumatic diseases might affect the heart. In their chapters, these authors attempt to define the state of the art of this topic.

The carotid artery is another conventional topic around ATS. Generally, the coronary circle is the first investigated system in patients with ATS and CAD. For this reason, we underline morbidity and mortality mainly related to carotid ATS instead of CAD.

A chapter dedicated to terminology analyzes old and new insights in order to better describe ATS manifestations, complications, and so on. New evidence needs new accurate and specific terminology, and general physicians, cardiologists, geriatricians, and other specialists involved with ATS must use the proper terms in managing and providing new treatments.

Finally, given the growing focus on gender medicine, a chapter on ATS and women explores the differences of the disease among men and women.

I would like to thank my team for collaborating on this book and bringing it to fruition. In particular, I am grateful to Bruno (my expert colleague) and Aurel (my secretary) for analyzing and reading the manuscript; Vincenzo, Stefano, and Andrea for evaluating the book's language; and Rebecca (my future wife) for sustaining me in all professional activities, giving me power in daily life!

Luigi Gianturco
ASST Rhodense, Cardio Rehab, Passirana-Rho Hospital,
Italy

Chapter 1

Introductory Chapter: Atherosclerosis, Arteriosclerosis, and Arteriolosclerosis

Luigi Gianturco

1. Background

Atherosclerosis (ATS) is still a great worldwide enemy despite the reduction of deaths due to it in the last two decades. Especially in Western countries, mortality was reduced thanks to anti-smoking laws. It is well established that smoking habits may accelerate ATS injury. Unfortunately, ATS morbidity and mortality are still high. Nowadays, the major cardiovascular (CV) risk (CVR) factors contributing to ATS are "metabolic": dyslipidemia, diabetes, and metabolic syndrome. That said, we understand how global CV disease (CVD) still determines about 30% of world deaths and ATS is definitely a pivotal contributor of CVD. For this reason, in literature, we have a multitude of papers about ATS.

2. General considerations

Let us summarize what is ATS: the term atherosclerosis refers to a generic hardening and loss of elasticity of the walls of the arteries for the formation of plaques, called atheromas or atherosclerotic plaques. Initially, they made up of lipids, including cholesterol, present in the blood and over time they tend to become getting bigger until developing a sort of "support structure" also composed of fibrous substances and connective cells. The latter, in the most advanced stage of the disease, calcify and degenerate going toward necrosis.

ATS can develop over the decades in silence, without giving any symptoms. When the first signs appear, generally after 40 years of age, the situation of the arteries is usually already compromised and the risk of complications, even serious ones, becomes very high.

ATS is often considered an exclusively cardiac problem, when in fact it can affect the arteries in any area of the body.

Normally ATS does not give symptoms until an artery is so narrowed or obstructed. Then, it would no longer be able to supply organs and tissues with an adequate blood flow. In these cases, you can witness manifestations similar to those of a myocardial infarction and/or stroke.

3. Treatment

Treatment of ATS involves, first of all, lifestyle correction (low-calorie and low-saturated fatty acid diet, exercise, smoking cessation), and pharmacological treatment of concomitant cardiovascular risk factors such as high blood pressure and diabetes mellitus. In some cases, when required by the guidelines, i.e., in secondary prevention and primary prevention in subjects with high cardiovascular risk, it is possible to resort to drugs that interact with the metabolism of cholesterol, such as statins, fenofibrates, or inhibitors of absorption cholesterol.

In selected cases and always if there are indications, it is possible to treat atherosclerotic lesions invasively with some surgical techniques. We know that angioplasty implants particular devices (stents) useful for keeping the lumen of the vessel dilated over time; the bypass that uses a blood vessel taken from another area of the body or implants a synthetic tube to allow blood to get around the artery and continue to flow. Furthermore, in case of thrombus, it is possible to implement a therapy that consists of injecting an anticoagulant drug into the affected tract to dissolve the thrombus and promote the outflow of blood.

Author details

Luigi Gianturco
ASST Rhodense, Cardio Rehab, Passirana-Rho Hospital, Italy

*Address all correspondence to: luigigianturco78@gmail.com

IntechOpen

Chapter 2

Carotid Disease

Minerva Irene Hernández Rejón
and Manuel Alexis Vargas Robles

Abstract

Atherosclerotic carotid disease causes about 30% of cerebrovascular ischemia transitory or permanent in the world; the severity of symptoms is variable. The clinical manifestations are varied from focal neurological alterations to transient or permanent vascular events. The treatment of the disease will depend on the location, degree, and risk, which can be surgical, endovascular, or medical. Open surgical treatment, endarterectomy, has been preferred as the first option and, however, has been reported to have associated complications like infection, hematoma, stroke, heart attack, restenosis, etc. With the advent of new technologies, endovascular treatment has been described as an option in patients with high risk or restenosis.

Keywords: atherosclerotic carotid disease, carotid endarterectomy, endovascular treatment, medical management of carotid disease, complications

1. Atherosclerotic disease and carotid stenosis

Atherosclerosis is a chronic disease of the arteries characterized by inflammation and plaque building in the arterial wall, eventually leading to stenosis of the vessel. Carotid atherosclerosis is associated with the increased risk of cardiovascular diseases [1].

Ischemic cardiovascular disease is a combination of progressive atherosclerosis and acute thrombotic complications [2].

The risk factors in atherosclerosis can be modifiable or not: non-modifiable are genetic predisposition, gender, and age, and modifiable factors are blood pressure, smoking, diabetes, cholesterol levels, obesity, and physical activity [2].

The earliest pathologic studies described the predilection of atherosclerosis near branch ostia, bifurcations, and bends, suggesting the important component of flow dynamics plays an important role in its initiation and development. Atherosclerotic plaque tends to form at regions where flow velocity and shear stress are reduced, in particular at the carotid bifurcation where disturbances in blood flow deviate from a laminar unidirectional pattern. Thus, the unique geometry and flow properties presented by the carotid bifurcation contribute [3].

Metabolic syndrome is a clinical entity characterized by multiple risk factors for cardiovascular disease and diabetes mellitus such as high-normal or elevated blood pressure, hyperglycemia, elevated triglycerides, low high-density cholesterol level, and abdominal obesity [4].

The increase of cardiovascular risk related to metabolic syndrome is reported; over the past decades, the impact of metabolic syndrome on large arterial vessels has been analyzed [4].

Carotid intima-media thickness has been proven to be a valuable predictor of myocardial infarction and ischemic stroke independent of traditional risk factor. The intima-media thickness was higher in patients with metabolic syndrome [4].

In the study IMPROVE, a multicenter observational European study, it showed that the intima-media thickness was a strong predictor of cardiovascular disease [4].

The maximum intima-media thickness of the common carotid artery, as measured by carotid artery ultrasound, has been used as a marker of atherosclerosis and cardiovascular disease. In contrast, there are reports suggesting that the predictive ability of intima-media thickness for cardiovascular disease is inferior than that of the carotid plaque score assessed by ultrasonography [5].

Recent studies have focused in adding pharmacological strategies like anti-thrombotic therapy, lowering lipid levels, improving glycemic control, and addressing inflammation present in the metabolic syndrome. On the other hand, patients with coronary and peripheral diseases have a high risk of cardiovascular death and disabling vascular events [2].

Carotid artery stenosis and lower limb peripheral arterial occlusive disease usually share the same pathological changes and can coexist. It has been reported that the prevalence rate of significant carotid stenosis increased with the stage of lower limb peripheral occlusive arterial disease. So the screening for significant carotid disease in these patients [6].

Screening for carotid stenosis in patients who are neurologically asymptomatic may therefore be acceptable when there are two or more risk factors or when ankle/brachial index is less than 0.4 with reevaluation of 6 months. Investigations have identified combinations of risks that identify populations in whom the risk of stenosis between 50% and 99% approaches 60%. Screening patients in these categories who are suitable operative candidates and who would undergo operation were the found to have clinically important disease [7].

2. Definition and epidemiology

Stroke diagnosis has been based on the World Health Organization's definition of a focal, occasionally global loss of neurological function lasting >24 h and which has a vascular etiology. A transient ischemic attack is defined in a similar way, but the duration is <24 h [8].

The principal causes of ischemic carotid territory stroke are thromboembolism from the internal carotid artery or middle cerebral artery (25%), small vessel intracranial disease (25%), cardiac embolism (20%), and other causes (5%). About 10–15% of all strokes follow thromboembolism from previously asymptomatic internal carotid stenosis >50% [9].

Moderate and severe carotid artery stenosis is an important public health issue; this condition affects 10% of the general population by their eighth decade and accounts for 10% of all strokes [10].

3. Clinical manifestations

The symptoms of the carotid disease were fist described by Fisher (1951). Stroke produced by carotid stenosis is caused by a combination of affection of the blood vessels, clotting system, and hemodynamics that in conjunction cause embolism or/and low cerebral flow [11].

Carotid atherosclerosis is usually most severe within 2 cm of the bifurcation of the common carotid artery and involving the posterior wall of the vessel. The definition of asymptomatic or symptomatic carotid artery stenosis is based on the history and physical examination [11].

Symptomatic symptoms include transient ischemic attacks produced by embolization that causes low flow with inadequate collateral blood supply. The symptoms depend on the cerebral artery territory involved, and total carotid artery occlusion can cause low flow or embolic ischemic events.

Various features of plaque morphology can be used to identify risk and include plaque ulceration, plaque structure and composition, and plaque volume [12].

A history of more than one episode of neurological alterations occurring in the same carotid territory is very suggestive of underlying carotid disease. The carotid bruit is an important sign over the site of the stenosis; however, is a poor predictor for development of stroke; and is not sufficiently predictive of high grade of carotid disease. However, 75% of patients with bruit had a moderate to severe stenosis (more than 60). Ischemic symptoms reflect ipsilateral ocular and cerebral hemisphere ischemia like partial or complete blindness, hemianopsia, hemiparesis, and hemisensory loss [12].

4. Diagnosis

There are four diagnostic modalities to directly image the internal carotid artery: cerebral angiography, carotid duplex ultrasound, magnetic resonance angiography, and computed tomography angiography.

Cerebral angiography is the gold standard for imaging the carotid arteries; it permits an evaluation of the entire carotid artery system, providing information about tandem atherosclerotic disease, plaque morphology, and collateral circulation; however, it is invasive, costs high, and has a high risk of morbidity and mortality [13].

There are three methods to measure carotid stenosis that predominate worldwide (NASCET, ECST, and CC):

- The North American Symptomatic Carotid Endarterectomy Trial (NASCET) measures the residual lumen diameter at the most stenotic portion and compares it with the normal internal carotid diameter [14].

- The European Carotid Surgery Trial (ECST) measures the lumen diameter at the most stenotic portion of the vessel and compares this with the estimated probable original diameter at the site of maximum stenosis [15].

- Common carotid (CC) measures the residual lumen diameter at the most stenotic portion of the vessel and compares this with the lumen diameter in the proximal common carotid artery [15].

Equivalent measurements for the three methods have been determined.

Carotid duplex ultrasound uses B-Mode to help detect focal increases in the blood flow velocity indicative of a high-grade carotid stenosis. The peak systolic velocity is the most frequently used measurement to gauge the severity of the stenosis (end-diastolic velocity, spectral configuration, and carotid index provide additional information) and correlate with the residual lumen diameter [16].

The sensitivity reported is 89% and the specificity 84%. It is a noninvasive, safe, and relative inexpensive technique, although it has limited utility in obtaining information about plaque composition and intraplaque hemorrhage and is less precise in determining stenosis of <50% compared with stenoses of higher degrees.

Transcranial Doppler is often used in conjunction with ultrasound carotid duplex to evaluate the hemodynamic significance of internal carotid artery stenosis [17].

Magnetic resonance angiography technique is used for evaluating the extracranial carotid arteries and produced a reproducible three-dimensional image of the carotid bifurcation with a good sensitivity for detecting high-grade carotid stenosis; however, it had been reported overestimated degree [18].

Computed tomography angiography provides an anatomic depiction of the carotid artery lumen, allows imaging of adjacent soft tissue structures, and is particularly useful when carotid duplex ultrasound is not reliable or when an overall view of the vascular field is required. It had a sensitivity and specificity of 97 and 99%, respectively [19].

In earlier reports, magnetic resonance, angiography, and carotid duplex ultrasound had difficulties distinguishing very severe stenosis from occlusion, so false-positive and false-negative results occurred [20].

The location most frequently affected by atherosclerosis is the carotid bifurcation. Progression of atheromatous plaque results in luminal narrowing, often accompanied by ulceration, process that can lead to ischemic stroke and transient ischemic attack from embolization, thrombosis, and hemodynamic compromise [20].

5. Treatment

5.1 Endarterectomy

The endarterectomy is the choice treatment in those patients with transient ischemic attacks or who suffered a cerebral infarction with a minimal sequel [21]. It is beneficial for symptomatic or asymptomatic patients.

The indications for carotid endarterectomy (CEA) are:

1. Bilateral carotid stenosis: in which the combined death and stroke rates in patients were almost twice than that of matched patients with unilateral disease (5.6% versus 2.4%) [22].

2. Prophylactic carotid endarterectomy: in patients with severe carotid stenosis prior to another surgery, it is rarely needed, and a decision to proceed should be individualized depending upon the clinician's best estimate of the risk of perioperative stroke.

3. Coronary artery bypass surgery: a new stroke or transient ischemic attack occurs in approximately 3% of patients following coronary artery bypass grafting (CABG); also in general surgery, the incidence of stroke appears to be lower in nonvascular surgical procedures than following cardiac surgery with a reported incidence in patients undergoing general anesthesia of less than 0.5%.

4. Vascular procedures: there are not enough trials for prophylactic CEA prior to abdominal aortic aneurysm repair or other major peripheral vascular procedures, because of the involvement of significant hemodynamic fluctuations.

5. Patients with intracranial aneurysm: ipsilateral intracranial aneurysms that are distal to a cervical internal carotid artery stenosis may be susceptible to sudden hemodynamic changes associated with CEA, leading to aneurysm rupture [23].

6. Contraindications for carotid endarterectomy

Absolute: asymptomatic complete carotid occlusion.

Relative contraindications: history of neck radiation, concurrent tracheostomy, prior radical neck dissection with or without radiation, contralateral vocal cord paralysis from prior endarterectomy, atypical lesion location, either high or low, that is surgically inaccessible, severe recurrent carotid stenosis, unacceptably high risk [24].

Carotid endarterectomy is established as safe and effective by randomized controlled trials for reducing the risk of ischemic stroke in both symptomatic and asymptomatic patients. However, carotid angioplasty and stenting are proposed as alternative for carotid endarterectomy.

Symptomatic carotid disease is defined as focal neurologic symptoms that are referable to the appropriate carotid artery distribution including transient ischemic attacks or ischemic strokes. The definition is contingent on the occurrence of carotid symptoms within the previous 6 months.

Carotid endarterectomy and stenting are recommended in patients with recently symptomatic carotid stenosis of 70–99% and a life expectancy of at least 5 years who meet all of these conditions: accessible carotid lesion, absence of clinically significant cardiac, pulmonary or other diseases that increase greatly the risk of anesthesia and surgery, and no prior ipsilateral endarterectomy.

It is suggested that carotid endarterectomy have to be done 2 weeks after a nondisabling stroke or transitory stroke, because between the first 48 hours, the risk of recurrent stroke elevates compared with later surgery. In patients who have a large infarction with brain swelling, hemorrhagic brain infarction and progressing stroke have long been thought to have high perioperative risk and expose the patient to an increased risk of recurrent stroke, emergent CEA for progressing/fluctuating stroke, or crescendo transitory attack that may have a high operative risk.

The risk of stroke can be calculated based on patient age, patient sex, degree of carotid stenosis, type of presenting symptomatic event, time since last symptomatic event, and carotid plaque morphology.

6.1 Surgical complications in carotid endarterectomy

Carotid endarterectomy complications can usually be related to comorbid conditions or cardiovascular preexisting diseases and also to the surgical technique. Most common complications of CEA include myocardial infarction, perioperative stroke, postoperative bleeding, and the potential consequences of cervical hematoma, nerve injury, surgical site infection, and carotid restenosis. However, the rates of complications after carotid endarterectomy is low [25–33].

There are two important trials in which the benefit is higher than the possible complications: the European Trial (ICSS) reports a mortality at 120 days of post-op of 0.8% and complications of 4.2%. The North American Trial (CREST) [33, 34] reported combined results for symptomatic and asymptomatic patients. In 1240 patients assigned to endarterectomy (47.3% asymptomatic), the 30-day death rate was 0.3%, and the rate of any periprocedural (30-day) stroke or death or postprocedural ipsilateral stroke was 2.3%.

Appropriate perioperative medication management is important to reduce the risk of cardiovascular and procedure-specific complications.

There are three mains risk factors:

1. Myocardial infarction

2. Stroke

3. Death

Others:

1. Hyperperfusion syndrome

2. Cervical hematoma

3. Nerve injury

4. Infection

5. Restenosis

There are a lot of risk factors, some of them are:

1. Age (>80 years)

2. Smoking

3. Previous stroke including transient ischemic attack

4. Previous stenosis of carotid artery

5. Special or chronic conditions such as cancer, heart diseases, hypertension, and diabetes

6.2 Myocardial infarction

In randomized trials, myocardial infarction has occurred at a slightly higher rate for carotid endarterectomy than carotid artery stenting [25, 26, 28–31]; with a reported incidence between 0 and 2%, pooled absolute risk of perioperative (30-day) myocardial infarction was 0.87%. The risk factors for myocardial infarction included older age, coronary heart disease, peripheral artery disease, and carotid restenosis.

6.3 Perioperative stroke

Perioperative stroke is the second most common cause of death in carotid endarterectomy [25, 26, 28, 32, 33, 35, 36] with a rate of less than 3% for symptomatic patients and less than 5% for the symptomatic patients depending on the indication of the CEA and the experience of the surgeon. But also there are some factors that can contribute to postoperative stroke [28, 37–42] like plaque emboli, platelet aggregates, improper flushing, poor cerebral protection, and relative hypotension.

If perioperative stroke is suspected, ultrasound is a good option; but if it shows good flow throughout the carotid artery with no thrombosis or intimal flaps, a head computed tomography (CT) scan should be obtained to rule out intracranial bleeding [38, 43–45]. If there is access to a hybrid operating room, another approach to obtain may be head CT first, and, if no bleeding is identified, intraoperative arteriography to identify any correctable lesions is performed [28].

6.4 Hyperperfusion syndrome

It is an uncommon complication of endarterectomy, occurring after carotid revascularization in less than 1%; it causes the most postoperative intracerebral hemorrhages and seizures in the first 2 weeks after CEA. It is caused after the surgery; because of the small vessels that chronically compensated the patient, and after endarterectomy blood flow is restored to a normal or elevated perfusion pressure and those vessels are unable to vasoconstrict sufficiently to protect the capillary bed, causing edema and hemorrhage and clinical manifestations. Hypertension is a frequent predecessor of the syndrome, underscoring the importance of good perioperative blood pressure control [46].

Hyperperfusion syndrome appears to be more likely with revascularization of a high-grade (80% or greater) stenosis.

Hyperperfusion syndrome is characterized by the following clinical features:

1. Headache ipsilateral to the revascularized internal carotid, typically improved in upright posture, may herald the syndrome in the first week after endarterectomy.

2. Focal motor seizures are common, sometimes with postictal Todd's paralysis mimicking post-endarterectomy stroke from carotid thrombosis.

3. Intracerebral hemorrhage is the most feared complication, occurring in approximatelys 0.6% of patients after CEA, usually within 2 weeks of surgery.

Treatment consists of prevention, strict control of postoperative hypertension maintaining a systolic blood pressure below 150 mmHg, and using labetalol, nitroprusside, and nitroglycerin aggressively. If complication is suspected in any patient with severe headache following CAE, a head CT is required to confirm or discard this syndrome [46, 47].

6.5 Cervical hematoma

This is a catastrophic and real urgent complication, because it can result in abrupt loss of the airway, with an incidence of 4% after CAE and requiring a re-exploration of the neck. Uncontrolled hypertension during emergence from anesthesia or in the postoperative period can also lead to hematoma formation [26, 35, 48].

6.6 Nerve injury

Cranial nerve or other nerve injuries occur in approximately 5% of patients following carotid endarterectomy [27, 33].

According to the European Carotid Surgery Trial, cranial nerve injury rate declined to 3.7%. In the Vascular Study Group of New England (VSGNE) database, the overall rate of nerve injury at discharge was 5.6%; 0.7% of patients had more than one nerve affected.

Hypoglossal nerve is the most frequently injurie manifested by a deviation of the tongue to the side of the injury, the facial nerve is the second one resulting in paresis of the lateral aspect of the orbicularis oris muscle with asymmetric smile; and the vagus nerve which result in unilateral vocal cord paralysis, glossopharyngeal nerve can be damaged with excessive dissection in the carotid bifurcation [26, 32, 36].

Injury to the sympathetic nerves can result in Horner's syndrome or, rarely, an entity called "first bite syndrome." Horner's syndrome can be complete (miosis, ptosis, anhidrosis) or partial (no anhidrosis) [29].

First bite syndrome is characterized by unilateral pain in the parotid region after the first bite of each meal felt to be due to sympathetic denervation of the parotid gland.

6.7 Infection

Surgical site/patch infection (SSI) rarely occurs following carotid endarterectomy, and, when they occur, most are superficial and self-limiting with antibiotic treatment. The prophylaxis is the best practice to prevent SSI.

Clinically the patient will have neck swelling and drainage from incision in acute events; in delayed infections, a draining sinus tract or pulsatile neck mass could be indicative of a carotid pseudoaneurysm. If infection persists, a patch excision is indicated with early carotid ligation, reconstruction with autogenous vein, or bypass; nowadays the use of negative pressure systems is a good option to perform a better treatment of these infections, resulting in better outcomes and reducing complications of a new exploratory surgery in these patients [3, 13, 19, 25–41].

6.8 Carotid restenosis

The pathology of the restenotic lesion is related to the time of presentation after initial surgery. Most patients with restenosis are asymptomatic and are identified with routine follow-up carotid imaging [29].

It is called early restenosis in those that occur within 2–3 years after CEA and late in those that occur more than 2–3 years after surgery. Patients at increased risk for restenosis include those below age 65, smokers, and women. Patch angioplasty appears to be associated with a decreased risk of long-term recurrent stenosis compared with primary closure [29, 31].

Reintervention is indicated in patients who develop neurologic symptoms referable to the carotid artery and those with restenosis >80% [29, 45].

6.9 Endovascular treatment

Carotid artery angioplasty and stenting are the standard for endovascular carotid intervention that is preferred for most patients with symptomatic internal carotid atherosclerosis. Patients with symptomatic carotid disease treated by endarterectomy that are considered to be less invasive have long-term benefits; nevertheless, it is reported that patients have an increased risk for poor outcomes with endarterectomy such as stroke periprocedural (30 days). So it is recommended in patients with 70–99% stenosis with the following conditions: not suitable surgical access, stenosis radiation induced, restenosis after endarterectomy, and clinically significant cardiac, pulmonary, or other disease that increment risk.

Low dose of aspirin treatment is recommended for all patients who are having an endarterectomy and have to be continued for at least 3 months after surgery; posterior only is indicated with cardiovascular disease.

The endovascular treatment is nowadays the first-line treatment for many vascular diseases. The percutaneous intraluminal angioplasty (PTA) consists in dilatation with a balloon for stenotic lesions, making a dehiscence effect, leading to fracture and separation of the arterial media from the intima; it was the first performed endovascular treatment. The introduction of stents was a major step in the evolution of the endovascular management of carotid stenosis [49].

There are a lot of diapositives that can be used in the endovascular treatment [22, 41, 50]; some of them are the following:

1. Cryoplasty is a type of balloon angioplasty that has liquid nitrous oxide to get inflated and uses cooling a-10°C (14°F) and pressure to dilate the plaque and vessel wall. It is well studied in iliac, infrainguinal, femoropopliteal, and popliteal lesions.

2. Focal pressure balloon was designed to reduce dissection and restenosis and to exhibit focal pressure to the lesions; it is used in infrapopliteal lesions.

3. Drug-coated balloon: drug-eluting stents (DES) achieve local administration of an agent capable of inhibiting intimal hyperplasia without systemic side effects. Cypher stents release sirolimus which has a potent immunosuppressive drug that controls intimal hyperplasia. TAXUS is a second-generation DES, with greater durability and which reduces restenosis. These devices are used in femoropopliteal lesions.

4. Stents are a method to reduce the incidence of restenosis or address balloon PTA failure due to elastic recoil or dissection. They are classified as balloon-expanding (BES) and self-expanding stents and also either as bare metal or covered stents. Self-expanding stents are composed typically of nitinol.

5. Stent grafts

   a. Balloon-expanding stent grafts can be expanded beyond the stated stent diameter; they are used for tracheobronchial strictures but not for PAD, for iliac or renal artery vascular beds, for occlusive lesions, as well as for perforation after PTA or stenting.

   b. Self-expanding stent grafts are used for various applications and in femoropopliteal disease and biliary applications.

   c. Drug-eluting stents have been associated with improved patency for the treatment of PAD compared to conventional balloon angioplasty. These are loaded with paclitaxel and sirolimus usually using polymers; these are used for femoropopliteal disease.

   d. Multilayer stents:

      i. Multilayer flow modulator (MFM) is designed to exclude peripheral or visceral aneurysm while maintaining branch vessel flow. It is a three-dimensional braided tube composed of multilayer wire without any covering prostheses.

      ii. Bioabsorbable stents are initially developed for coronary intervention, now is used also for peripheral arterial beds.

Author details

Minerva Irene Hernández Rejón* and Manuel Alexis Vargas Robles
Department of General Surgery, Hospital Central Norte PEMEX, Mexico City,
Mexico

*Address all correspondence to: minehdezr@gmail.com

IntechOpen

References

[1] Forgo B, Medda E, Hernyes A, Szalontai L, Tarnoki DL, Tarnoki AD. Carotid artery atherosclerosis: A review on heritability and genetics. Twin Research and Human Genetics. 2018:1-14

[2] Vanassche T, Verhamme P, Anand SS, Shestakovska O, Fox KAA, Bhatt DL, et al. Risk factors and clinical outcomes in chronic coronary and peripheral artery disease: An analysis of the randomized, double-blind COMPASS trial. European Journal of Preventive Cardiology. 2019;27(3):296-307

[3] Kolodgie FD, Nakazawa G, Sangiorgi G, Ladich E. Pathology of atherosclerosis and stenting. Neuroimaging Clinics of North America. 2009;17(3):1-25

[4] Cuspidi C et al. Metabolic syndrome and subclinical carotid damage: A meta-analysis from population-based studies. Journal of Hypertension. 2017;36:1-8

[5] Kawada T, Andou T, Fukumitsu M. Metabolic syndrome showed significant relationship with carotid atherosclerosis. Heart and Vessels. 2015;31(5):664-670

[6] Pan Z, Wang R, Li L, Zhang H. Correlation between significant asymptomatic carotid artery stenosis and severity of peripheral arterial occlusive disease in the lower limb: A retrospective study on 200 patients. BMC Neurology. 2019:4-8

[7] Cina CS, It SC, Safar HA. Prevalence and progression of internal carotid artery stenosis in patients with peripheral arterial occlusive disease. Journal of Vascular Surgery. 2000;36(1): 75-82

[8] Abbott AL. Optimizing the definitions of stroke, transient ischemic attack, and infarction for research and application in clinical practice. Frontiers in Neurology. 2017;8(October):1-14

[9] Persoon S, Kappelle LJ, Klijn CJM. Limb-shaking transient ischaemic attacks in patients with internal carotid artery occlusion: A case-control study. Brain: A Journal of Neurology. 2010

[10] Vranic H, Hadzimehmedagic A, Haxibeqiri-karabdic I. Critical carotid artery stenosis in coronary and non-coronary patients—Frequency of risk factors. Medical Archives. 2017;71(2): 110-114

[11] Witteman JCM, Grobbee DE, Hofman A, Breteler MMB. Carotid plaques increase the risk of stroke and subtypes of cerebral infarction in asymptomatic elderly the rotterdam study. Circulation. 2002:2872-2877

[12] Takaya N, Yuan C, Chu B, Saam T, Underhill H, Cai J, et al. Subsequent ischemic cerebrovascular events a prospective assessment with MRI—Initial results. Stroke. 2006;112:818-823

[13] Hankey GJ, Warlow CP, Sellar RJ. Cerebral angiographic risk in mild cerebrovascular disease. Stroke. 1990: 209-222

[14] Commite S. Original contributions North American symptomatic carotid endarterectomy trial. Stroke. 1991

[15] James F, Toole JEC. Accurate measurement of carotid stenosis. American Society of Neuroimaging. 1994

[16] Polak F, Leary HO. Detection and carotid artery various Doppler quantification of stenosis: Efficacy of velocity parameters. AJR. 1993;160: 619-625

[17] Edwards JM et al. Correlation of North American Symptomatic Carotid

Endarterectomy Trial (NASCET) angiographic definition of 70% to 99% internal carotid artery stenosis with duplex scanning. Journal of Vascular Surgery. 1993

[18] Bowen C, Pattany M, Quencer M. Review article MR angiography head and neck: Of occlusive disease current concepts of the arteries in the. AJR. 1994:9-18

[19] Corti R, Ferrari C, Roberti M, Alerci M, Pedrazzi PL, Gallino A. Spiral computed tomography A novel diagnostic approach for investigation of the extracranial cerebral arteries and its complementary role in duplex ultrasonography. Circulation. 1998:984-989

[20] Mattle HP, Kent KC, Edelman R. Evaluation of the extracranial carotid arteries: Correlation of magnetic resonance angiography , duplex ultrasonography, and conventional angiography. Journal of Vascular Surgery. 1991;**13**(6):838-845

[21] Seara AH. Tratamiento quirúrgico de la estenosis carotídea [Surgical treatment of the carotid stenosis]. 2014;**15**(2):153-170

[22] Counsell CE, Salinas R, Naylor R, Warlow CP. A systematic review of the randomised trials of carotid patch angioplasty in carotid endarterectomy. European Journal of Vascular and Endovascular Surgery. 1997;**13**(4):345-354

[23] Da Silva AF, Mccollum P, Szymanska T, De Cossart L. Prospective study of carotid endarterectomy and contralateral carotid occlusion. The British Journal of Surgery. 1996;**83**(10):1370-1372

[24] Marcucci G, Accrocca F, Antonelli RG, Giordano A, Gabrielli R, Mounayergi F, et al. High-risk patients for carotid endarterectomy: Turned

down cases are rare. Journal of Cardiovascular Surgery. 2012;**53**:333-343

[25] Boulanger M, Camelière L, Felgueiras R, Berger L, Rerkasem K, Rothwell PM, et al. Periprocedural myocardial infarction after carotid endarterectomy and stenting: Systematic review and meta-analysis. Stroke. 2015;**46**(10):2843-2848

[26] Texakalidis P, Giannopoulos S, Charisis N, Giannopoulos S, Karasavvidis T, Koullias G, et al. A meta-analysis of randomized trials comparing bovine pericardium and other patch materials for carotid endarterectomy. Journal of Vascular Surgery. 2018;**68**(4):1241-1256.e1

[27] Kragsterman B, Björck M, Wanhainen A. EndoVAC, a novel hybrid technique to treat infected vascular reconstructions with an endograft and vacuum-assisted wound closure. Journal of Endovascular Therapy. 2011;**18**(5):666-673

[28] Krafcik BM, Cheng TW, Farber A, Kalish JA, Rybin D, Doros G, et al. Perioperative outcomes after reoperative carotid endarterectomy are worse than expected. Journal of Vascular Surgery. 2018;**67**(3):793-798

[29] Rambachan A, Smith TR, Saha S, Eskandari MK, Bendok BR, Kim JYS. Reasons for readmission after carotid endarterectomy. World Neurosurgery. 2014;**82**(6):E771-E776

[30] Bennett KM, Kent KC, Schumacher J, Greenberg CC, Scarborough JE. Targeting the most important complications in vascular surgery. Journal of Vascular Surgery. 2017;**65**(3):793-803

[31] Enomoto LM, Hill DC, Dillon PW, Han DC, Hollenbeak CS. Surgical specialty and outcomes for carotid endarterectomy: Evidence from the

National Surgical Quality Improvement Program. The Journal of Surgical Research. 2014;**188**(1):339-348

[32] Rizzo A, Hertzer NR, O'Hara PJ, Krajewski LP, Beven EG. Dacron carotid patch infection: A report of eight cases. Journal of Vascular Surgery. 2000;**32**(3):602-606

[33] Ederle J, Dobson J, Featherstone RL, Bonati LH, van der Worp HB, de Borst GJ, et al. Carotid artery stenting compared with endarterectomy in patients with symptomatic carotid stenosis (International Carotid Stenting Study): An interim analysis of a randomised controlled trial. Lancet. 2010;**375**(9719):985-997

[34] Clark WM, Brooks W, Mackey A, Hill MD, Leimgruber PP, Sheffet AJ, et al. New England Journal. 2010:11-23

[35] Ho KJ, Nguyen LL, Menard MT. Intermediate-term outcome of carotid endarterectomy with bovine pericardial patch closure compared with Dacron patch and primary closure. Journal of Vascular Surgery. 2012;**55**(3):708-714

[36] Fatima J, Federico VP, Scali ST, Feezor RJ, Berceli SA, Giles KA, et al. Management of patch infections after carotid endarterectomy and utility of femoral vein interposition bypass graft. Journal of Vascular Surgery. 2019;**69**(6):1815-1823.e1

[37] Acosta S, Björck M, Wanhainen A. Negative-pressure wound therapy for prevention and treatment of surgical-site infections after vascular surgery. The British Journal of Surgery. 2017;**104**(2):e75-e84

[38] Hammer FD. Reply. Journal of Vascular Surgery. 2001;**33**(3):662-663

[39] Inui T, Bandyk DF. Vascular surgical site infection: Risk factors and preventive measures. Seminars in Vascular Surgery. 2015;**28**(3-4):201-207

[40] Muto A, Nishibe T, Dardik H, Dardik A. Patches for carotid artery endarterectomy: Current materials and prospects. Journal of Vascular Surgery. 2009;**50**(1):206-213

[41] Rangel-Castilla L, Rajah GB, Shakir HJ, Davies JM, Snyder KV, Siddiqui AH, et al. Endovascular prevention and treatment of stroke related to extracranial carotid artery disease. The Journal of Cardiovascular Surgery. 2017;**58**(1):35-48

[42] Perler BA, Ursin F, Shanks U, Williams GM. Carotid dacron patch angioplasty: Immediate and long-term results of a prospective series. Vascular. 1995;**3**(6):631-636

[43] Hyldig N, Birke-Sorensen H, Kruse M, Vinter C, Joergensen JS, Sorensen JA, et al. Meta-analysis of negative-pressure wound therapy for closed surgical incisions. The British Journal of Surgery. 2016;**103**(5):477-486

[44] Stone PA, Srivastava M, Campbell JE, Mousa AY, Hass SH, Kazmi H, et al. A 10-year experience of infection following carotid endarterectomy with patch angioplasty. Journal of Vascular Surgery. 2011;**53**(6):1473-1477

[45] van der Slegt J, Kluytmans JAJW, de Groot HGW, van der Laan L. Treatment of surgical site infections (SSI) IN patients with peripheral arterial disease: An observational study. International Journal of Surgery. 2015;**14**:85-89

[46] Hosoda K, Kawaguchi T, Ishii K, Minoshima S, Shibata Y, Iwakura M, et al. Prediction of hyperperfusion after carotid endarterectomy by brain SPECT analysis with semiquantitative statistical mapping method. Stroke. 2003;**34**(5):1187-1193

[47] Kablak-Ziembicka A, Przewlocki T, Pieniazek P, Musialek P, Tekieli L, Rosławiecka A, et al. Predictors of

cerebral reperfusion injury after carotid stenting: The role of transcranial color-coded doppler ultrasonography. Journal of Endovascular Therapy. 2010;**17**(4):556-563

[48] Illuminati G, Calio' FG, D'Urso A, Ceccanei G, Pacilè MA. Management of carotid Dacron patch infection: A case report using median sternotomy for proximal common carotid artery control and in situ polytetrafluoroethylene grafting. Annals of Vascular Surgery. 2009;**23**(6):786.e1-786.e5

[49] Eller JL, Snyder KV, Siddiqui AH. Endovascular treatment of carotid stenosis. Neurosurgery Clinics of North America. 2014;**25**(3):565-582

[50] Bederson JB, Sander Connolly E Jr, Batjer HH, Dacey RG, Dion JE, Diringer MN, et al., American Heart Association. Guidelines for the management of aneurysmal subarachnoid hemorrhage: A statement for healthcare professionals from a special writing group of the stroke council, American heart association. Stroke. 2009;**40**(3):994-1025

Intermittent Hypoxia and Obstructive Sleep Apnea: Mechanisms, Interindividual Responses and Clinical Insights

Lena Lavie

Abstract

Obstructive sleep apnea (OSA), a nightly respiratory condition, is characterized by recurrent upper airway collapse causing intermittent hypoxia (IH) resembling ischemia and reperfusion (I/R). Consequently, blood oxygenation levels are cyclically reduced; sleep fragmentation and sympathetic activation develop, thus invoking oxidative stress and inflammation. OSA is a major risk factor for cardio-/cerebrovascular morbidity and mortality. However, not all OSA patients develop cardio-/cerebrovascular disease, even if suffering from similar OSA severity. Possibly, this results from interindividual differences in responses to a given hypoxic stimulus involving gene polymorphism in oxygen-regulated transcription factors and downstream genes. The current review is aimed at highlighting potentially protective mechanisms induced by IH and OSA, rather than its well-established deleterious effects, while focusing on acute coronary syndromes. Therefore, protective mechanisms revealed in I/R biology and exhibited in vitro and in animal models utilizing IH followed by a severe ischemia are discussed and linked to acute myocardial infarction patients with concomitant OSA. The roles of endothelial progenitor cells, their proliferative and angiogenic properties, and collateral formation are emphasized in the clinical setting, as well as heterogenic interindividual responses to identical hypoxic stimuli. These findings might represent potential predictors to cardio-/cerebrovascular health, by identifying patients at higher or lower cardiovascular risk.

Keywords: intermittent hypoxia, hypoxia, endothelial progenitor cells (EPCs), endothelial cell colony-forming units (EC-CFUs), endothelial tube formation, hypoxia-inducible factor (HIF)-1α, vascular endothelial growth factor (VEGF), coronary collaterals

1. Introduction

Obstructive sleep apnea (OSA) is a nightly respiratory condition characterized by recurrent oropharyngeal upper airway collapse during sleep leading to multiple cycles of hypoxic episodes followed by blood reoxygenation. While blocking the respiratory system in OSA provokes hypoxic events, resuming respiration induces the reoxygenation phase. This intermittent respiration results in multiple cycles of hypoxia and reoxygenation throughout the night which are termed intermittent hypoxia (IH). This intermittent respiration directly affects blood oxygenation/ deoxygenation levels altering physiological biochemical and molecular pathways [1].

The significance of OSA to human health stems from its high prevalence worldwide, the complaints regarding the quality of life, and the association with cardiovascular and other comorbidities. It is identified by a loud and intermittent snoring, excessive daytime sleepiness, and polysomnographic respiratory findings. In the general population with classical complaints, as loud snoring and excessive daytime sleepiness, OSA affects 4 and 2% of adult men and women particularly after menopause, respectively. However, these values are much higher in the general population not having the classical complaints and are estimated to be as high as 24% in men and 9% in women. Moreover, in selected populations like the obese and the elderly, this value may rise up to 60% [1, 2]. Moreover, OSA is a well-established cardiovascular and cerebrovascular risk. It is currently implicated in the etiopathogenesis of cardiovascular comorbidities, arrhythmias, congestive heart failure, hypertension, atherosclerosis, and stroke [1].

Intermittent hypoxia is in fact the hallmark of OSA. Consequently, many physiological, cellular, and biochemical alternations occur due to the cyclically reduced blood oxygenation levels, sleep becomes fragmented, and sympathetic nerve activity develops [3]. The severity of the IH and the hypoxemia in OSA are determined by the number of the hypoxic events per hour of sleep, termed Apnea-Hypopnea Index (AHI). It mostly ranges from a cutoff point of 10 events per hour of sleep for normal breathing to mild (11–20), moderate (21–30), and severe OSA (>30 events per hour of sleep). In severe patients, blood oxygenation levels can intermittently drop to as low as 60%.

Events of IH in OSA and in animal models treated with IH were shown to elicit cell and tissue injury by increasing the formation of reactive oxygen species (ROS) and promoting inflammatory pathways. Both oxidative stress and inflammation are fundamental mechanisms in various pathologies, inducing vascular dysfunction, transcriptional reprograming, inflammation, and innate and adaptive immune activation, all of which are contributors of morbidity and mortality in a vast array of cardiovascular and other morbidities [4]. This sequence of events initiated by IH is illustrated in **Figure 1**, which was adapted from Lavie [3] and published by Levy et al. [1].

To date, the deleterious effects of OSA and IH on the cardio-/cerebrovascular system are well established, many of which result from the IH-associated oxidative stress, systemic inflammation, and sympathetic nerve activation. These fundamental components are largely responsible for inducing endothelial dysfunction and vascular comorbidities in these patients [1, 3]. Specifically, IH was shown to induce activation of various leukocyte subpopulations, by increasing their ROS and inflammatory cytokine production. Moreover, increased expression of adhesion molecules, increased avidly of OSA monocytes to endothelial cells, inhibition of neutrophil apoptosis, and increased cytotoxicity of CD8+ T lymphocytes and γδ T cells toward endothelial cells were also shown to contribute to endothelial cell damage, as illustrated in **Figure 1** [3, 5–7]. Thus, the multiple cycles of IH in OSA have been shown to resemble mechanisms of ischemia and reperfusion (I/R) injury by eliciting similar fundamental mechanisms, including increased ROS production, activated leukocytes, inflammation, transcriptional reprograming, and vascular dysfunction [5, 6, 8].

Importantly, although the most prominent and notable effects of I/R reveal tissue and organ injury leading to cardiovascular and cerebrovascular morbidity, I/R was also shown to confer cardioprotection by activating adaptive mechanisms such as ischemic preconditioning (IPC), post-conditioning, and remote-conditioning [9]. Thus, since not all OSA patients develop cardiovascular and other morbidities, it is feasible that in some instances IPC may occur in OSA as well. Apparently, genetic polymorphism in HIF-1 and downstream genes as vascular endothelial growth factor (VEGF) and erythropoietin (EPO) might influence the individual responses to a given IH stimulus. However, also environmental- and lifestyle-related variables (diet, sports, air pollution) could affect these individual responses [1, 3].

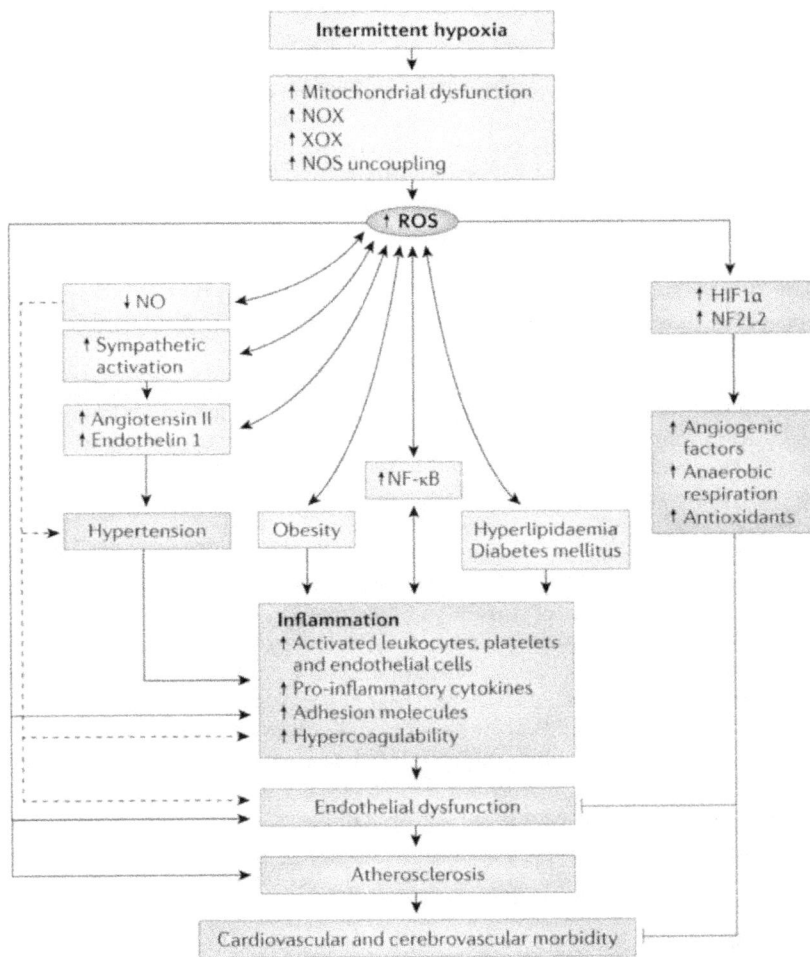

Figure 1.
Oxidative stress promotes sympathetic activation, cellular and systemic inflammation, and vascular comorbidities in OSA. Intermittent hypoxia induces the production of reactive oxygen species (ROS), resulting in oxidative stress by inducing mitochondrial dysfunction, activating NADPH oxidase (NOX) and xanthine oxidase (XOX), and inducing nitric oxide synthase (NOS) uncoupling. Interaction of ROS with nitric oxide (NO) further promotes oxidative stress while diminishing the bioavailability of NO and thus promoting hypertension, inflammation, endothelial dysfunction, hypercoagulability, and atherosclerosis. The ROS-dependent increase in sympathetic activation and in angiotensin II and endothelin 1 levels contribute to hypertension. Concomitantly, ROS can upregulate numerous redox-sensitive transcription factors, such as nuclear factor-κB (NF-κB), hypoxia-inducible factor-1α (HIF-1α), and nuclear factor (erythroid-derived 2)-like 2 (NF2L2). NF-κB orchestrates the various inflammatory processes that lead to endothelial dysfunction and atherosclerosis. By contrast, HIF-1α and NF2L2, which are also upregulated by ROS levels, are involved in protective mechanisms, which may counteract some of deleterious effects of ROS. Comorbidities and conditions associated with OSA, such as hypercholesterolemia, diabetes mellitus, and obesity, also have a ROS component and involve NF-κB activation and inflammation. Broken line, indirect pathway; red line, inhibition. Figure adapted from Ref. [3], Elsevier and published in Lévy et al. [1].

The current review is aimed at highlighting potentially protective mechanisms induced by IH and OSA rather than the deleterious and well-established injurious effects described above while focusing on OSA patients with concomitant acute coronary syndromes. Thus, protective mechanisms revealed in I/R biology and also exhibited in animal models of IH after a global ischemic insult, as well as in patients with acute myocardial infarction (AMI) and concomitant OSA, are discussed and further elaborated in models of IH in vitro. A special emphasis is put on endothelial progenitor cells (EPCs), their proliferative and angiogenic properties, and their association with collateral formation. The significance of the heterogeneity in the proliferative and angiogenic functions of EPCs from healthy individuals exposed to a given identical IH stimulus is discussed with regard to potential collateral development and cardiovascular outcomes. Understanding individual differences to various forms of hypoxia and the associated molecular pathways can help in identifying patients at higher or lower cardiovascular risk.

2. Protective mechanisms associated with ischemia and reperfusion

The preconditioning effect is basically an experimental strategy. Applying brief ischemic episodes each followed by reperfusion—prior to a longer and potentially lethal duration of ischemia—can confer protection to an organ or a tissue. IPC of the heart is the best studied one. It demonstrates the heart's own self-preserving mechanism, by reducing infarct size and ventricular arrhythmias, and was shown in many of the models studied. In the first and seminal study demonstrating IPC [10], dog hearts were preconditioned by undergoing four circumflex coronary occlusions each lasting 5 min, separated each by 5 min of reperfusion (a total of 40 min), followed by a sustained 40 min occlusion and 4 days of reperfusion recovery. Control animals underwent only a single 40 min of occlusion and 4 days of reperfusion recovery after which infarct size was measured. In the controls, the infarcted area consisted 30% of the area at risk, whereas that of the preconditioned animals was only 7.5% of the area at risk (25% of the infarct size in the controls). This landmark study has paved the way to subsequent studies demonstrating the protective effects of IPC in the kidney, brain, liver, and intestine [11, 12]. Moreover, in various studies, the paradigms of IPC varied considerably ranging from intervals of minutes to seconds. Thus, when nonlethal sequential episodes of I/R—like those occurring in OSA nightly, prior to the occurrence of an acute lethal I/R episode—like in AMI or stroke, preconditioning may occur in those patients.

2.1 Mechanisms of ischemic preconditioning in animal models of intermittent hypoxia

The mechanisms involving IPC are complex and intricate, implicating various molecular, cellular, and paracrine pathways. Some of the triggers, mediators, and targets activated by I/R include Ca^{+2} ions, ROS, reactive nitrogen species, purinergic signaling, kinases, cytokines, and mitochondria. Transcriptional reprograming is affected as well. It involves upregulation of the redox-sensitive transcription factor hypoxia-inducible factor (HIF)-1α and its downstream genes VEGF and EPO and inducible nitric oxide synthase (iNOS) [4, 12]. The angiogenic VEGF promotes neovascularization and collateral vessel formation, while EPO is essential for protection against I/R injury. Nuclear factor kB (NF-κB) and some of its regulated inflammatory pathways are activated as well. Collectively, these transcriptional alterations invoke cellular and paracrine functions. In that context, a number of studies utilizing animal models of IH were shown to reduce infarct size in rat hearts and improve focal ischemic injury in mice. In an acute model of IH, isolated rat myocardium was exposed to 4 h or 30 min of preconditioning by IH, using hypoxic episodes of either 10 or 5% oxygen, lasting 40 s and normoxia at 21% O_2 for 20 s (60 IH events per hour). After 24 h of recovery, sustained ischemia lasting 30 min was followed by 120 min of reperfusion. Only the paradigm of 4 h of IH at 10% oxygen induced a delayed preconditioning by reducing infarct size to more than 50% as compared to control hearts [13]. Moreover, besides reducing infarct size, also HIF-1α was stabilized and iNOS was activated. These effects were mediated through PKC and triggered by P38 MAPK and ERK1/ERK2 while inhibiting iNOS with aminoguanidine before the ischemic period abolished the IPC phenomenon [14]. In a chronic IH model investigating focal ischemic injury in mice, a dichotomous effect was noted. The mice were subjected to chronic IH at 10 or 6% O_2 for 35 days (8 h/day 20 hypoxic episodes/hour lasting 90 s at 90 s of intervals) or to room air (sham). Then the mice were treated for focal ischemic injury for 30–35 min. Only at 10% of O_2, EPO and VEGF were increased, while inflammatory markers were decreased compared to controls. At the more severe IH of 6% of O_2, inflammatory markers were increased as compared to control sham animals [15]. In both the acute and the chronic IH animal models described, the IH served as a nonlethal preconditioning effect before applying the lethal I/R stimulus. Acute as well as chronic IH displayed dichotomous effects, depending on the severity of the IH applied. Moreover, the molecular mechanisms described for IH-dependent IPC concur with classical IPC mechanisms in I/R (upregulation of HIF-1α, VEGF, EPO, and iNOS). Thus, the protective effects were dependent on the severity, the frequency, and the chronicity of the IH paradigms applied in these animal models of IH.

2.2 Potential involvement of IPC in OSA patients with acute MI and acute ischemic stroke

The involvement of IPC is potentially implicated in patients with OSA after an AMI or an acute ischemic stroke. For instance, peak cardiac troponin values were shown to be significantly higher in AMI patients without OSA than in AMI patients with OSA. This finding suggests that OSA might have a protective effect in the context of MI and that patients with OSA may experience less severe myocardial injury [16]. Additionally, the prevalence of non-ST-elevation myocardial infarction (NSTEMI) in AMI patients was associated with OSA and was shown to increase with the increasing severity of OSA. This finding may also suggest a cardioprotective role of OSA, which may attenuate the development of ST-elevation myocardial infarction (STEMI), perhaps through IPC [17]. In patients with OSA hospitalized because of an acute ischemic stroke, less severe neurological injury and lower unadjusted mortality rates were found than in those without a history of OSA [18]. Also, cardiac arrest survivors with OSA had better unadjusted survival rates and favorable adjusted neurological outcomes at discharge than those without OSA [19]. This latter study suggests that OSA patients may tolerate better acute brain ischemia due to preconditioning. Collectively, these recent studies favor the possibility that the presence of OSA may confer cardio-/neuroprotection in patients with AMI or acute ischemic stroke.

3. The role of endothelial progenitor cells in endothelial health

Blood-derived EPCs play a pivotal role in maintaining vascular homeostasis by providing an endogenous repair mechanism by replacing dysfunctional endothelium and enhancing tissue repair after an ischemic vascular insult [20, 21]. EPCs are mobilized by hypoxia or tissue ischemia, HIF-1α- and VEGF-dependent pathways [22].

In AMI patients, EPCs were shown to home at the ischemic myocardium and participate in vascular and cardiac repair, basically acting as an internal pool of endothelial cells (ECs). EPCs contribute up to 25% of ECs in newly developed vessels at ischemic sites. Hence, they promote coronary collateral formation while improving endothelial functions by integrating into newly developing capillaries or into injured blood vessels [20, 23]. Of note, low EPC numbers were shown to correlate with endothelial dysfunction, atherosclerosis, and poor cardiovascular outcome. Thus, they are currently considered in many studies to represent an independent predictor of endothelial dysfunction and long-term prognosis in patients with coronary artery disease [21, 24]. Therefore, circulating EPC levels might be used as a surrogate marker to assess clinical outcomes.

In most of the studies published thus far, EPCs were primarily identified by CD34 (primitive hematopoietic progenitors) and VEGF-R2 (a VEGF receptor) expressions [20]. Their proliferative and angiogenic capacities were demonstrated in vitro by two widely used assays: (1) the formation of endothelial colonies in culture—termed endothelial cell colony-forming units (EC-CFUs) [25]—and (2) the determination of the paracrine effects of these developed colonies on endothelial cells in culture [26].

Growing EPCs on fibronectin in vitro can induce proliferation and differentiation into EC-CFUs which are characterized by a central core of round angiogenic T cells and outgrowing spindle-shaped cells. These colonies secret angiogenic growth factors such as VEGF inducing endothelial tube formation via paracrine pathways. Moreover, in AMI patients the expression of circulating EPCs (CD34+/VEGF-R2) was positively correlated with mean endothelial tube formation [27]. Also, EC-CFUs were shown to negatively correlate with the Framingham risk score, thus adequately representing circulating EPCs [25]. Both these two in vitro measures—the formation of EC-CFUs in culture and their paracrine effects on endothelial tube formation— might be considered as good surrogate markers for circulating EPCs [25, 27].

3.1 Endothelial progenitor cells and their proliferative and angiogenic properties in AMI patients with OSA

Acute MI can be a devastating I/R event and a frequent cause of sudden death. Sleep apnea is highly prevalent in AMI patients, ranging in various studies from 22 to 69%. However, in the setting of AMI, the presence of OSA is frequently not considered and therefore under diagnosed [28]. Evaluating circulating EPCs in patients diagnosed with OSA while recovering from an AMI revealed significantly higher EPC numbers than in AMI patients without OSA. Also the intracellular VEGF expression, EC-CFU numbers, and their angiogenic T cells in culture, and endothelial tube formation, were all significantly higher than those in AMI patients without OSA [27]. These findings suggest that the IH associated with OSA might have a crucial role in promoting these protective functions of EPCs in the setting of AMI. Subsequently, the development of EC-CFUs and their paracrine functions in healthy individuals were determined by exposure to IH in vitro. Indeed, the proliferative and paracrine abilities of EC-CFUs and endothelial tube formation were increased by IH, as compared to those that developed under normoxic conditions [27, 29]. Moreover, IH in vitro increased NADPH oxidase-dependent ROS production, protein carbonylation, and VEGF expression in EC-CFUs. Both EC-CFU numbers and endothelial tube formation in culture were increased by ROS-dependent mechanisms. Accordingly, ROS scavengers and NADPH oxidase inhibitors attenuated or completely abolished the formation of EC-CFUs treated by IH in vitro. It is therefore likely that IH and ROS are crucial contributors to increased EPC numbers and their proliferative and angiogenic functions [29].

4. Development of coronary collaterals in acute coronary syndromes

A number of studies demonstrate that coronary collaterals were increased in coronary artery disease patients with high EPC numbers. Conversely, inadequate coronary collateral development was associated with reduced numbers of circulating EPCs and impaired pro-angiogenic activity, as determined by the low values of EC-CFUs and tube formation in culture [30, 31]. Moreover, increased circulating EPC levels were also associated with collateral formation in patients with NSTEMI [32]. Furthermore, reduced circulating EPC numbers also predicted future cardiovascular events, emphasizing the clinical importance of endogenous vascular repair [30, 31, 33]. Therefore, circulating EPC numbers might represent a good prognostic marker for the outcomes in the clinical context of acute coronary syndrome [20].

Interestingly in OSA patients with total coronary occlusion, collateral development was significantly higher than in non-OSA patients with the same coronary occlusion (Rentrop score 2.4 ± 0.7 vs. 1.61 ± 1.2, $p = 0.02$, respectively) [34]. Similar finding supporting increased coronary collaterals in inaugural AMI patients with OSA was also reported more recently [35].

5. Interindividual responses to hypoxic conditions

Interindividual differences are fundamental to the development of personalized medicine. Different individuals respond in a distinctively different manner to an identical hypoxic stimulus. Such diverse responses can result from a number of reasons. Specifically, however, genetic variations in the expression of oxygen-regulated genes are of a particular interest in this growing field of personalized and regenerative medicine, as EPCs and their proliferative and angiogenic functions are [3]. For instance, the expression of the transcription factor HIF-1α and some of its downstream genes as VEGF and aldolase C was determined in lymphocytes from healthy adults exposed to eight different hypoxic treatments ranging from 0.1 to 20% oxygen. The sensitivity of HIF-1α expression to hypoxia varied considerably between individuals. HIF expression in the "low responders" was upregulated at 0.1% oxygen, whereas "high responders" upregulated HIF already at 5% oxygen. Moreover, also the HIF-regulated downstream genes responded in the same manner in each individual, suggesting that the source of this variation resides within the HIF system itself [36]. Furthermore, in patients with ischemic heart disease, DNA was genotyped for single-nucleotide polymorphism (C or T changes at residue 582 of HIF-1α, from proline to serine). HIF-1α polymorphism was associated with the development of collaterals in those patients and was dependent on the frequency of the T alleles. Its frequency was higher in patients without collaterals than in patients with collaterals (the presence of CT or TT was a negative predictor). Thus, variations in HIF-1α genotype may influence the development of collaterals in patients with significant coronary artery disease perhaps regardless of the severity of the ischemia they encounter [37]. In an earlier study, interindividual responses to hypoxia were also shown in coronary artery disease patients undergoing angiography. Their monocytes were harvested and exposed to an identical hypoxic stimulus. Then, mRNA levels of VEGF were determined and correlated with the presence of collaterals. Patients with no collaterals had significantly lower hypoxic induction of mRNA VEGF levels, whereas high mRNA VEGF levels were correlated with high collateral formation [38]. Collectively, these latter studies emphasize the heterogenic responses observed between different individuals exposed to an identical hypoxic stimulus, due to a different genetic background. Moreover, the significance of collateral development in the context of individual responses and clinical outcomes is further emphasized.

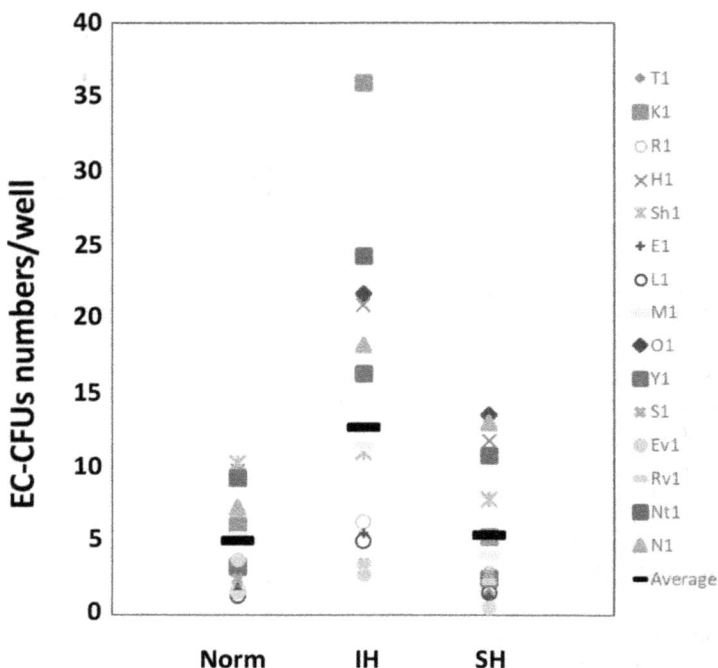

Figure 2.
Individual and mean EC-CFU numbers were determined on the 7th day in culture in 15 healthy donors. Cells were exposed to intermittent hypoxia (IH) and to sustained hypoxia (SH) and compared to normoxia (Norm). Each symbol represents a different donor. The horizontal black bar represents the average value for each treatment. (IH 12.7 ± 10.0 vs. Norm 5.0 ± 3.3 EC-CFUs/well, p < 0.017; SH 5.4 ± 4.7 vs. Norm EC-CFUs/ well, p = NS). These data were published in Avezov et al. [29].

Since high levels of EC-CFUs and endothelial tube formation were correlated with high collateral formation [30, 31], we investigated the effects on EC-CFUs, endothelial tube formation, and VEGF levels in young healthy adults by applying IH in vitro. As aforementioned, IH increased the formation of EC-CFUs and their paracrine activity by increasing endothelial tube formation via higher VEGF expression in culture [29]. However, there was also a significant variation within the cellular responses to the hypoxic stimuli between individuals as depicted in **Figure 2**. This latter finding emphasizes again the importance of the interindividual heterogeneity observed in the hypoxic responses to a specific stimulus as described earlier for the HIF system and the downstream genes in cardiovascular patients as well as in healthy individuals [36–38].

6. Conclusions

Intermittent hypoxia is the hallmark of obstructive sleep apnea. However, many of the molecular pathways activated in OSA and in response to IH in vivo and in vitro resemble pathways activated by ischemia and reperfusion (I/R). This is evident in injurious as well as in protective mechanisms. IH, similar to I/R, promotes fundamentally injurious mechanisms as oxidative stress and inflammation which invoke atherosclerotic processes rendering OSA a major risk factor for cardio- and cerebrovascular disease. Yet, not all OSA patients develop these morbidities. Importantly, also, similar to I/R, some OSA patients with concomitant acute MI respond to the harsh effects of IH by activating akin molecular pathways which promote protective mechanisms as ischemic preconditioning. It is therefore likely that OSA promotes IPC in some instances as well. This is particularly evident in patients recovering from AMI.

Both IH and ROS were shown to play a major role in increasing EPC and EC-CFU numbers and angiogenic functions. All in all, circulating EPC numbers and their angiogenic functions were shown to represent a good surrogate marker as well as a prognostic marker to assess the outcomes in the clinical context of acute MI. This is emphasized by their association and significance to collateral development and clinical outcome. Moreover, the heterogenic responses observed between individuals, implicating a specific personal response to a given particular stimulus, based on genetic variants, might be considered as the foundation for developing personalized medicine for acute MI patients. Thus, IH might be considered as a new modality for the upregulation of angiogenic processes to induce collateral formation in the clinical setting. However, the severity, the frequency, and the chronicity of the IH paradigms should be determined in order to identify and harness IH patterns possessing protective effects. Collectively, based on the studies presented in this review, it is clearly evident that determination of collateral formation, EPC numbers (and possibly their proliferative and angiogenic properties), HIF polymorphism, downstream genes as VEGF, and additional markers, yet to be unraveled, represent an important tool to identify patients at higher or lower risk for outcomes of acute coronary syndromes. However, no less important is the identification of IH patterns possessing protective effects toward elevating EPC numbers in the circulation of acute MI patients with low or unfavorable HIF polymorphism.

Acknowledgements

Drs. Slava Berger and Katia Avezov are gratefully acknowledged for their insightful findings. The Guzik Foundation, USA, is gratefully acknowledged for their generous support.

Conflict of interest

None to declare.

Author details

Lena Lavie
The Lloyd Rigler Sleep Apnea Research Laboratory, Unit of Anatomy and Cell Biology, The Ruth and Bruce Rappaport Faculty of Medicine, Technion-Israel Institute of Technology, Haifa, Israel

*Address all correspondence to: lenal@technion.ac.il

IntechOpen

References

[1] Levy P, Kohler M, McNicholas WT, Barbe F, McEvoy RD, Somers VK, et al. Obstructive sleep apnoea syndrome. Nature Reviews. Disease Primers. 2015;1:15015. DOI: 10.1038/nrdp.2015.15

[2] Punjabi NM. The epidemiology of adult obstructive sleep apnea. Proceedings of the American Thoracic Society. 2008;5:136-143. DOI: 10.1513/pats.200709-155MG

[3] Lavie L. Oxidative stress in obstructive sleep apnea and intermittent hypoxia—Revisited—The bad ugly and good: Implications to the heart and brain. Sleep Medicine Reviews. 2015;20:27-45. DOI: 10.1016/j.smrv.2014.07.003

[4] Eltzschig HK, Eckle T. Ischemia and reperfusion—From mechanism to translation. Nature Medicine. 2011;17:1391-1401. DOI: 10.1038/nm.2507

[5] Dyugovskaya L, Lavie P, Lavie L. Increased adhesion molecules expression and production of reactive oxygen species in leukocytes of sleep apnea patients. American Journal of Respiratory and Critical Care Medicine. 2002;165:934-939. DOI: 10.1164/ajrccm.165.7.2104126

[6] Dyugovskaya L, Lavie P, Lavie L. Phenotypic and functional characterization of blood gammadelta T cells in sleep apnea. American Journal of Respiratory and Critical Care Medicine. 2003;168:242-249. DOI: 10.1164/rccm.200210-1226OC

[7] Dyugovskaya L, Polyakov A, Cohen-Kaplan V, Lavie P, Lavie L. Bax/Mcl-1 balance affects neutrophil survival in intermittent hypoxia and obstructive sleep apnea: Effects of p38MAPK and ERK1/2 signaling. Journal of Translational Medicine. 2012;10:211. DOI: 10.1186/1479-5876-10-211

[8] Lavie L. Obstructive sleep apnoea syndrome—An oxidative stress disorder. Sleep Medicine Reviews. 2003;7:35-51. DOI: 10.1053/smrv.2002.0261

[9] Hausenloy DJ, Yellon DM. The therapeutic potential of ischemic conditioning: An update. Nature Reviews Cardiology. 2011;8:619-629. DOI: DOI 10.1038/nrcardio.2011.85

[10] Murry CE, Jennings RB, Reimer KA. Preconditioning with ischemia: A delay of lethal cell injury in ischemic myocardium. Circulation. 1986;74:1124-1136. https://doi.org/10.1161/01.CIR.74.5.1124

[11] Stokfisz K, Ledakowicz-Polak A, Zagorski M, Zielinska M. Ischaemic preconditioning—Current knowledge and potential future applications after 30 years of experience. Advances in Medical Sciences. 2017;62:307-316. DOI: 10.1016/j.advms.2016.11.006

[12] Heusch G. Molecular basis of cardioprotection: Signal transduction in ischemic pre-, post-, and remote conditioning. Circulation Research. 2015;116:674-699. DOI: 10.1161/CIRCRESAHA.116.305348

[13] Beguin PC, Joyeux-Faure M, Godin-Ribuot D, Levy P, Ribuot C. Acute intermittent hypoxia improves rat myocardium tolerance to ischemia. Journal of Applied Physiology. 2005;99:1064-1069. DOI: 10.1152/japplphysiol.00056.2005

[14] Belaidi E, Beguin PC, Levy P, Ribuot C, Godin-Ribuot D. Prevention of HIF-1 activation and iNOS gene targeting by low-dose cadmium results in loss of myocardial hypoxic preconditioning in the rat. American Journal of Physiology. Heart and Circulatory Physiology. 2008;294:H901-H908. DOI: 10.1152/ajpheart.00715.2007

[15] Jackman KA, Zhou P, Faraco G, Peixoto PM, Coleman C, Voss HU, et al. Dichotomous effects of chronic intermittent hypoxia on focal cerebral ischemic injury. Stroke. 2014;**45**:1460-1467. DOI: 10.1161/STROKEAHA.114.004816

[16] Sanchez-de-la-Torre A, Soler X, Barbe F, Flores M, Maisel A, Malhotra A, et al. Cardiac troponin values in patients with acute coronary syndrome and sleep apnea: A pilot study. Chest. 2018;**153**:329-338. DOI: 10.1016/j.chest.2017.06.046

[17] Ludka O, Stepanova R, Sert-Kuniyoshi F, Spinar J, Somers VK, Kara T. Differential likelihood of NSTEMI vs STEMI in patients with sleep apnea. International Journal of Cardiology. 2017;**248**:64-68. DOI: 10.1016/j.ijcard.2017.06.034

[18] Festic N, Alejos D, Bansal V, Mooney L, Fredrickson PA, Castillo PR, et al. Sleep apnea in patients hospitalized with acute ischemic stroke: Underrecognition and associated clinical outcomes. Journal of Clinical Sleep Medicine. 2018;**14**:75-80. DOI: 10.5664/jcsm.6884

[19] Alejos D, Festic E, Guru P, Moss JE. Neurological outcomes of patients with history of obstructive sleep apnea after a cardiac arrest. Resuscitation. 2017;**119**:13-17. DOI: 10.1016/j.resuscitation.2017.07.027

[20] Leal V, Ribeiro CF, Oliveiros B, Antonio N, Silva S. Intrinsic vascular repair by endothelial progenitor cells in acute coronary syndromes: An update overview. Stem Cell Reviews. 2018;**15**:35-47. DOI: 10.1007/s12015-018-9857-2

[21] Rigato M, Avogaro A, Fadini GP. Levels of circulating progenitor cells, cardiovascular outcomes and death: A meta-analysis of prospective observational studies. Circulation Research. 2016;**118**:1930-1939. DOI: 10.1161/CIRCRESAHA.116.308366

[22] Cuadrado-Godia E, Regueiro A, Nunez J, Diaz-Ricard M, Novella S, Oliveras A, et al. Endothelial progenitor cells predict cardiovascular events after atherothrombotic stroke and acute myocardial infarction. A PROCELL substudy. PLoS One. 2015;**10**:e0132415. DOI: 10.1371/journal.pone.0132415

[23] Asahara T, Takahashi T, Masuda H, Kalka C, Chen D, Iwaguro H, et al. VEGF contributes to postnatal neovascularization by mobilizing bone marrow-derived endothelial progenitor cells. The EMBO Journal. 1999;**18**:3964-3972. DOI: 10.1093/emboj/18.14.3964

[24] Werner N, Wassmann S, Ahlers P, Schiegl T, Kosiol S, Link A, et al. Endothelial progenitor cells correlate with endothelial function in patients with coronary artery disease. Basic Research in Cardiology. 2007;**102**:565-571. DOI: 10.1007/s00395-007-0680-1

[25] Hill JM, Zalos G, Halcox JP, Schenke WH, Waclawiw MA, Quyyumi AA, et al. Circulating endothelial progenitor cells, vascular function, and cardiovascular risk. The New England Journal of Medicine. 2003;**348**:593-600. DOI: 10.1056/NEJMoa022287

[26] Bauer J, Margolis M, Schreiner C, Edgell CJ, Azizkhan J, Lazarowski E, et al. In vitro model of angiogenesis using a human endothelium-derived permanent cell line: Contributions of induced gene expression, G-proteins, and integrins. Journal of Cellular Physiology. 1992;**153**:437-449. DOI: 10.1002/jcp.1041530302

[27] Berger S, Aronson D, Lavie P, Lavie L. Endothelial progenitor cells in acute myocardial infarction and sleep-disordered breathing. American Journal of Respiratory and Critical Care Medicine. 2013;**187**:90-98. DOI: 10.1164/rccm.201206-1144OC

[28] Aronson D, Nakhleh M, Zeidan-Shwiri T, Mutlak M, Lavie P,

Lavie L. Clinical implications of sleep disordered breathing in acute myocardial infarction. PLoS One. 2014;**9**:e88878. DOI: 10.1371/journal.pone.0088878

[29] Avezov K, Aizenbud D, Lavie L. Intermittent hypoxia induced formation of "Endothelial Cell-Colony Forming Units (EC-CFUs)" is affected by ROS and oxidative stress. Frontiers in Neurology. 2018;**9**:447. DOI: 10.3389/fneur.2018.00447

[30] Lambiase PD, Edwards RJ, Anthopoulos P, Rahman S, Meng YG, Bucknall CA, et al. Circulating humoral factors and endothelial progenitor cells in patients with differing coronary collateral support. Circulation. 2004;**109**:2986-2992. DOI: 10.1161/01.CIR.0000130639.97284.EC

[31] Matsuo Y, Imanishi T, Hayashi Y, Tomobuchi Y, Kubo T, Hano T, et al. The effect of endothelial progenitor cells on the development of collateral formation in patients with coronary artery disease. Internal Medicine. 2008;**47** 127-134. DOI: JST.JSTAGE/internalmedicine/47.0284

[32] Lev EI, Kleiman NS, Birnbaum Y, Harris D, Korbling M, Estrov Z. Circulating endothelial progenitor cells and coronary collaterals in patients with non-ST segment elevation myocardial infarction. Journal of Vascular Research. 2005;**42**:408-414. DOI: 10.1159/000087370

[33] Schmidt-Lucke C, Rossig L, Fichtlscherer S, Vasa M, Britten M, Kamper U, et al. Reduced number of circulating endothelial progenitor cells predicts future cardiovascular events: Proof of concept for the clinical importance of endogenous vascular repair. Circulation. 2005;**111**:2981-2987. DOI: 10.1161/CIRCULATIONAHA.104.504340

[34] Steiner S, Schueller PO, Schulze V, Strauer BE. Occurrence of coronary collateral vessels in patients with sleep apnea and total coronary occlusion. Chest. 2010;**137**:516-520. DOI: 10.1378/chest.09-1136

[35] Ben Ahmed H, Boussaid H, Longo S, Tlili R, Fazaa S, Baccar H, et al. Impact of obstructive sleep apnea in recruitment of coronary collaterality during inaugural acute myocardial infarction. Annales de Cardiologie et d'Angéiologie. 2015;**64**:273-278. DOI: 10.1016/j.ancard.2015.01.014

[36] Brooks JT, Elvidge GP, Glenny L, Gleadle JM, Liu C, Ragoussis J, et al. Variations within oxygen-regulated gene expression in humans. Journal of Applied Physiology (Bethesda, MD: 1985). 2009;**106**:212-220. DOI: 10.1152/japplphysiol.90578.2008

[37] Resar JR, Roguin A, Voner J, Nasir K, Hennebry TA, Miller JM, et al. Hypoxia-inducible factor 1alpha polymorphism and coronary collaterals in patients with ischemic heart disease. Chest. 2005;**128**:787-791. DOI: 10.1378/chest.128.2.787

[38] Schultz A, Lavie L, Hochberg I, Beyar R, Stone T, Skorecki K, et al. Interindividual heterogeneity in the hypoxic regulation of VEGF: Significance for the development of the coronary artery collateral circulation. Circulation. 1999;**100**:547-552

Chapter 4

Atherosclerosis in Rheumatology: Old and New Insights

Sabina Oreska and Michal Tomcik

Abstract

Cardiovascular diseases are the leading cause of morbidity and mortality in general population worldwide. There is an increasing significance of cardiovascular risk in the field of rheumatology, and accordingly, the evidence on the relation between immune system disorders and atherosclerosis has been substantially growing especially in last decades. Since novel immune and metabolic factors are considered to participate in pathogenesis of atherosclerosis and increased cardiovascular risk in rheumatic patients, they are getting to the forefront of the research. Since novel therapeutic approaches have improved survival of rheumatic patients, and decreased morbidity caused by rheumatic disease activity and damage, the significance of other comorbidities leading to premature mortality has arisen. Nevertheless, appropriate recommendations for the management of cardiovascular risk are still lacking. Recently, European League Against Rheumatism (EULAR) recommendations for management of the cardiovascular risk and comorbidities in patients with inflammatory arthropathies have been published. However, the cardiovascular management of these patients is still suboptimal. In addition, the situation in other orphan diseases such as idiopathic inflammatory myopathies, systemic sclerosis and others is even more uncertain and strongly requires further research. This chapter provides an overview of epidemiology, pathogenesis, clinical manifestations, screening and management of atherosclerosis in patients with rheumatic diseases.

Keywords: atherosclerosis, rheumatic diseases, metabolic risk factors, management, therapy

1. Introduction

Cardiovascular diseases (CVDs) are estimated to be the leading cause of mortality and morbidity worldwide and are responsible for one-third of world's population mortality [1]. Atherosclerosis (ATS), as the main cause of CVD, starts to develop early in the life and presents later with clinical manifestations depending on other circumstances. ATS is a multifactorial disease, in which the immune system and impairment of vascular system play a significant role. Inflammation, which can be triggered by infectious agents or by autoimmune reaction, worsens and promotes atherogenesis by several mechanisms [2]. In addition to the immune system, other factors significantly participate in atherogenesis by facilitating the vascular damage, initiating the formation, progression and the rupture of atherosclerotic plaques leading to consequent clinical manifestation of ATS. So-called traditional risk factors include dysregulation of lipid and glucose metabolism, arterial hypertension, and degeneration of vascular tissue caused by aging, smoking and hormonal factors [3].

It is well known that autoimmune diseases are accompanied by increased CV morbidity and mortality, caused by exacerbation of atherogenesis [2]. Traditional risk factors of ATS in general population such as dyslipidemia, glucose intolerance, arterial hypertension, etc. can explain only about 75% of CV manifestations in rheumatic patients [4]. In these patients, non-traditional risk factors associated with the systemic inflammatory disease apply [5].

Despite the significant improvement of the therapy of rheumatic diseases, the incidence of CVD in rheumatic patients remains increased compared to that in general population [6]. Both the CV risk and CVD manifestations differ among rheumatic diseases according to the characteristic pathogenetic mechanism, inflammation activity and other specific features of the rheumatic diseases [7]. CV risk in the more prevalent rheumatic diseases such as rheumatoid arthritis (RA) or systemic lupus erythematosus (SLE) is relatively best described. On the other hand, the situation is less clear in orphan connective tissue diseases such as systemic sclerosis (SSc), idiopathic inflammatory myopathies (IIM), primary Sjögren's syndrome (pSS) and others.

The aim of this review chapter is to provide an overview and sum up the current knowledge on CV risk factors and the treatment options of ATS-related comorbidities in rheumatic diseases.

2. Cardiovascular risks in rheumatic diseases

Traditional CV risk factors play two roles in rheumatic patients: the first one as a trigger, the second as a consequence of the rheumatic disease activity [3]. Non-traditional risk factors are given by genetic and epigenetic factors, concurrent autoimmune inflammatory disorder and the specific features of each particular rheumatic disease (age of onset, duration, activity and the type of the disease) and other comorbidities, among others depression [8–10].

2.1 Metabolic syndrome and its association with immune disorders

Metabolic syndrome (MetS) is defined as a cluster of comorbidities and risk factors leading to CVDs and increasing the CV mortality and morbidity. MetS includes obesity and visceral adiposity, diabetes and insulin resistance (IR), arterial hypertension (AH) and dyslipidemia [11]. The matter of mutual interactions and cross-talk of immune and metabolic system has become the object of many studies in recent years. Immune-metabolic interactions are regulated by genetic factors, nutritional status and by intestinal microbiome. The imbalance of the immune and metabolic interactions contributes to the occurrence and manifestation of rheumatic diseases [12].

The prevalence of MetS in general population is estimated to be 24–44% depending on the exact definition of the MetS and the studied population [11, 13], and increases in rheumatic patients and gout to as much as 36–42%, as was reported in studies comparing rheumatic patients to the healthy control population [13].

Different immune mechanisms have been reported to be implemented in the pathogenesis of MetS, including pro-inflammatory cytokines, namely interleukin (IL)-1 and IL-12 family. These cytokines are included in the regulation of immune response and atherogenic damage, and in the differentiation of T helper cells (Th), which participate in the pathogenesis of both autoimmune disorders and CVDs [14, 15]. Cytokines of IL-23/IL-17 signaling pathway are increased in rheumatic diseases, and significantly participate in atherogenesis [16]. MetS is associated with increased oxidative stress, which, among others, leads to the formation of oxidized phospholipids (oxPL) and contributes to pathogenesis of autoimmune disorders [13].

IR is not only closely related to MetS, but is also considered to act as a key pathogenic factor in MetS [13]. The definition describes IR as a decreased sensitivity and responsiveness of target organs to the action of insulin resulting in hyperinsulinemia [17]. As consequence, this metabolic disorder leads to glucotoxicity, lipotoxicity and inflammation, all of which participate in endothelial damage and dysfunction [18]. The visceral fat tissue is considered to be the major locus of these unfavorable changes. Of note, CVDs, MetS and autoimmune disorders share common pathogenic mechanisms and mediators of inflammation and activity [13].

In recent years, study of microbiome has come to the forefront of interest. An imbalance of intestinal microbiota (dysbiosis) is characterized by a decrease of the number of beneficial intestinal bacteria and the overgrowth of potentially pathogenic bacteria. This phenomenon accompanies metabolic disorders and contributes to the emergence of MetS, obesity and type 2 diabetes mellitus (T2DM) [19]. Impaired balance of the intestinal flora may also contribute to the development of autoimmune disorders. Several studies have demonstrated onset of inflammation induced by alterations in the gut microbiome. This could explain the relationship between the microbiome and systemic inflammatory response [20].

2.2 Obesity as an active contributor to inflammation

The definition of obesity is mostly based on the body mass index (BMI—values higher than 30 kg/m^2). Obesity, as well as MetS, is a global health problem especially in developed countries. The prevalence has been constantly growing over the years and to date, it is estimated to be almost 40% in the general population [21, 22]. Nevertheless, the association of obesity and CVDs in the general population is not clear [23]. Some evidence even suggests better prognosis for people with higher value of BMI [24]. However, there is a well-known correlation of obesity and increased risk of T2DM and coronary arterial disease (CAD), as well as a negative impact of obesity on other comorbidities including rheumatic diseases [23]. The immunomodulatory potential of adipose tissue and its ability to create an inflammatory environment of moderate activity could explain the effect of obesity as a risk factor for the development of some autoimmune diseases [22, 25].

Adipose tissue not only consists of adipocytes and connective tissue cells, but also contains immune cells as well (T cells, eosinophils, B regulatory cells and macrophages) [26–28]. In individuals with normal BMI, the immune cells interact with adipocytes and maintain a non-inflammatory environment by production of anti-inflammatory cytokines (IL-10, IL-4, IL-13) [27]. On the contrary, predominance of pro-inflammatory T helper (Th) type 1 and 17 cells and pro-inflammatory type of macrophages has been found in increased adipose tissue mass of obese individuals [27, 29, 30]. These changes result in the production of pro-inflammatory molecules such as tumor necrosis factor (TNF) and IL-6, which are one of the crucial cytokines involved in the pathogenesis of several rheumatic diseases. Moreover, obesity leads to an altered expression of adipokines, multifunctional molecules produced by white adipose tissue cells and involved in the regulation of inflammatory and autoimmune processes [31, 32]. The MetS and secretion of pro-inflammatory adipokines can be associated with CVDs and autoimmune disorders [13].

Thus, obesity is not only a passive comorbidity, but can actively participate in the inflammatory process. According to the current evidence, obesity can negatively affect the course of most rheumatic diseases, functional disability, quality of life and the overall prognosis [21, 22].

2.3 Dyslipidemia in autoimmune disorders

Dyslipidemia is one of the most common forms of metabolic disease in the general population and also a significant risk factor for atherogenic CVD. In the general population, dyslipidemia is characterized by an increased level of total cholesterol (TC), low-density lipoproteins (LDLs), triglycerides (TGs) and a decreased level of high-density lipoproteins (HDLs) [33]. Under normal circumstances, HDL (in normal serum levels) exerts an anti-atherogenic effect: it removes cholesterol particles from cells (especially macrophages in the artery wall) and from circulation; inhibits the migration of macrophages and the binding of monocytes to the endothelium, oxidation of LDL; promotes endothelial repair and improves endothelial function, and also exerts anti-inflammatory and anti-apoptotic effects [34–36]. In systemic inflammation, HDL is converted into a dysfunctional form due to loss of anti-inflammatory and anti-oxidative proteins. The modification of apolipoprotein A1 (apo-A1) results in the inability of HDL to uptake LDL from macrophages and in the activation of pro-inflammatory pathways leading to increased risk of coronary artery involvement [35, 37].

Moreover, quantitative changes of lipidogram related to disease activity are often seen in rheumatic diseases. In RA patients, the levels of TC and LDL are lower than in general population. This so-called lipid paradox, best described in RA, is associated with an increased CV risk [37]. Decrease in levels of TC and LDL has been found to precede clinical manifestation of RA. Later, TC and LDL levels tend to increase after the initiation of immunosuppressive therapy and on the contrary, decline during the relapse of RA [38]. Therefore, the low levels of TC and LDL can be misinterpreted as a low CV risk factor when evaluated according to the scoring tools (e.g., Framingham risk score, Reynolds risk score, Systemic Coronary Risk Evaluation—SCORE) [39–41].

A small study in early RA patients reported non-significant, beneficial effect of methotrexate similar to that of tumor necrosis factor inhibitors (anti-TNF) on lipidogram [42]. On the other hand, higher levels of TC, LDL and TG were described in patients with ankylosing spondylitis (AS) treated by anti-TNF compared to AS patients on nonsteroidal anti-inflammatory drug (NSAID) therapy. Nevertheless, results reported in a cross-sectional study do not allow for a generalized assessment of the influence of long-term anti-TNF therapy on lipidogram in AS [43].

Dyslipidemia is found in almost half of SLE patients, characterized by elevated levels of very-low density lipoprotein (VLDL) and TG. Increased levels of TC and TG are associated with two times increased risk of CVD [44]. In SSc, dyslipidemia is characterized by increased levels of lipoprotein A (LpA) and LDL and decreased levels of HDL and TC [45].

2.4 Role of immune system and autoantibodies in atherogenesis

The presence of immune cells in atherosclerotic plaques proves the participation of immune system in atherogenesis [46, 47]. These infiltrating immune cells are responsible for the promotion and exacerbation of ATS [48]. All the components of immune system are included in atherogenesis, while TNF and IL-1β are the most significant pro-inflammatory cytokines and mediators [1].

Damage of endothelium is the first step in atherogenesis. Particles circulating in the blood penetrate the damaged endothelial barrier into subendothelial layer via the interaction with adhesion molecules on the surface of endothelium. These reactions lead to activation of endothelium and attraction of immune cells [1]. Penetrating particles consist mainly of LDL, which are one of the targets of oxidation and form oxLDL (oxidized LDL). oxLDLs are taken up by macrophages, which subsequently transform into the foam cells. Specific autoantibodies against oxLDL (anti-oxLDL) were detected in the sera of individuals from the general population as well as in rheumatic patients [49]. Furthermore, in rheumatic patients, the levels of anti-oxLDL are increased compared to those in the general population [49, 50]. The presence of these antibodies can predict the peripheral vascular involvement and even the severity of ATS [51]. On the other hand, increased levels of anti-oxLDL antibodies in patients with pSS were paradoxically associated with decreased occurrence of plaques (unlike in RA or SLE), which suggests a possible protective role of anti-oxLDL antibodies in pSS [52].

Many autoantibodies have been described to have a relation to higher risk of ATS and its clinical manifestations [2]. These include the antibodies against heat shock proteins (HSPs), which are expressed on the surface of endothelial cells exposed to stress, and to β-2-glycoprotein I (β2GPI), which are abundantly expressed within the subendothelial layer and intima-media borders of plaques [46, 53]. Furthermore, antinuclear antibodies (ANAs) are more frequently detected in patients with symptomatic angina pectoris and the three-vessel disease compared to individuals without coronary artery involvement [54]. Moreover, ANA positivity is associated with an increased risk of myocardial infarction (MI) in non-rheumatic individuals [55]. Specific anti-endothelial cell antibodies (AECAs) are associated with subclinical or manifested ATS in non-rheumatic population, as well [56].

2.5 Immunosuppressive therapy and its effect on CV risk

Immunosuppressive therapy of rheumatic diseases has a potential effect on CV morbidity and mortality in two ways: on the one hand, it suppresses the inflammatory activity and thus decreases the CV risk; on the other hand, the adverse effect of some drugs can worsen the CV risk [9, 57]. NSAIDs and coxibs (selective blockers of cyclooxygenase-2) mostly used in inflammatory arthropathies exert pro-thrombotic effect and have a negative impact on the CV risk. Due to this fact, benefit-risk ratio should be evaluated individually in every case. Naproxen is considered as the relatively safest drug from this group [58].

Corticosteroids (CSs) suppress the inflammatory activity, hence dampen the CV risk [59, 60]. On the other hand, CSs cause or worsen the traditional CV risk factors [61]. Meta-analysis evaluating CS therapy in RA reported that a long-term therapy with prednisone or prednisone-equivalents in high doses (above 7.5 mg per day) is associated with an increased risk of CV mortality [62]. The effect of lower doses (7.5–10 mg a day) is uncertain [63]. Duration and the cumulative dose of CS are considered as CV risk factors in SLE. Nevertheless, current evidence regarding the CS therapy in SLE is not conclusive [44]. European League Against Rheumatism (EULAR) recommends, especially in inflammatory arthropathies, to keep the glucocorticoid dosage to a minimum and to taper glucocorticoids in case of remission or low disease activity and to regularly check the reasons to continue glucocorticoid therapy [59].

The group of disease-modifying anti-rheumatic drugs (DMARDs) is a heterogeneous entity of medicaments with immunosuppressive effects of various specificity: less specific conventional synthetic DMARDs (csDMARD), or more specific biologic (bDMARDs), biosimilar (bsDMARDs) or targeted synthetic molecules (tsDMARDs). The side effects differ within the whole group. csDMARDs have a potential to reduce atherogenesis and progression of ATS [64]. Thus, the early initiation of therapy with scDMARDs can prevent development of CVDs [65].

Antimalarial drugs have been reported to act favorably on lipid and glucose metabolism, and in SLE patients, they have been described to reduce hypercholesterolemia, ATS and the risk of thrombosis [44, 66, 67]. In addition, hydroxychloroquine (HCQ) influences the production of cytokines, activation of T cells and monocytes via interaction with Toll-like receptor (TLR) signaling pathway, and attenuates the oxidative stress and endothelial dysfunction [68].

The effects of methotrexate (MTX) on the CV risk have been best studied in RA, in which the potential to reduce the risk of heart failure by half was demonstrated [69]. Moreover, MTX can decrease the mortality of RA patients caused by CVDs by 30% [70]. The data suggest that MTX should be considered cardioprotective in rheumatic diseases, although the exact mechanism of this effect is not known yet [71]. A possible link with anti-inflammatory effect has been proposed [72]. On the other hand, according to the results of a recent randomized controlled trial in patients with carotid artery disease or history of MI and concurrent T2DM or MetS, no protective effect of MTX in low doses (15–20 mg weekly) on future risk of CVD was described [73]. Data in other DMARDs are insufficient and, therefore, the effect on CV risk is not clear.

bDMARDs are targeting selectively specific pro-inflammatory molecules, which significantly participate in both pathogenesis of inflammatory diseases and atherogenesis (e.g., TNF, IL-1r, IL-6 and others) [74]. In this group, TNF inhibitors (anti-TNFs) are the best-studied drugs regarding the possible effect on the CV risk. On the one hand, they exert anti-inflammatory and anti-atherogenic effect; on the other hand, they have been demonstrated to worsen the cardiac insufficiency in a couple of first published studies [3, 8]. Their benefit was proven in several randomized controlled trials (RCTs) with more or less significantly beneficial effect when compared to MTX [72, 75–77]. Anti-TNFa influences particularly the level of HDL and restores its anti-atherogenic potential [78]. The results of RCTs in RA, PsA and psoriasis show a beneficial effect of anti-TNF therapy on glucose metabolism and MetS [79]. Anti-TNFs also reduce the risk of T2DM manifestation and prevent endothelial damage due to specific inhibition of TNF [74, 80]. Overall, current data support the beneficial effect of anti-TNF therapy on CV risk and CVD incidence that is probably related to the attenuation of inflammation and thus also of atherogenesis rather than to the effect on lipidogram (which can change as a consequence of changes in disease activity as well). Published studies have reported the potential of anti-TNF to reduce intima-media thickness and the number of unstable plaques [81]. Nevertheless, anti-TNF therapy is not recommended in patients with congestive heart failure [82]. Not only no positive effect, but even a negative effect of anti-TNF on chronic heart failure has been described. Experts therefore suggest performing a baseline echocardiography examination in patients at risk before the commencement of anti-TNF therapy [81].

Higher IL-6 levels are associated with an increased CV risk, therefore therapeutic blockade of tocilizumab (inhibitor of IL-6 receptor) has a protective potential [83]. Recently published RCT with tocilizumab and etanercept (anti-TNF) reported very similar effect of both drugs on CV risk [84]. Inhibition of the IL-6 receptor by tocilizumab is assumed to influence lipid metabolism in a favorable manner due to blockade of the mobilization of fatty acids to peripheral tissues mediated by IL-6 [84]. On the contrary, anti-IL-6r therapy is known to cause a significant increase in the levels of HDL, TC, LDL and TG [85].

Rituximab (RTX, anti-CD20) is supposed to have a beneficial effect on CV risk due to inhibition of B cells and release of (auto)antibodies, which participate in the vasoconstriction, activation of thrombocytes and promote rupture of atherosclerotic plaques [74]. In SLE patients, the RTX therapy was associated with improvement of lipidogram [86]. The overall effect of RTX on CV risk is not clear, due to limited data and lack of SLE patients treated by RTX [44]. To date, studies with RTX have not shown any long-term adverse cardiovascular effects or cardiotoxicity [74, 87].

The recent study CANTOS (Canacinumab Antiinflammatory Thrombosis Outcome Study) has proven the ability of anti-IL-1b (canacinumab) to reduce the CV events and stroke in non-rheumatic patients with history of MI [88]. The effect of bDMARDs, including the latest bsDMARDs and tsDMARDs, on the CV risk needs to be closely monitored and evaluated in long-term studies with sufficiently large cohorts of rheumatic patients.

3. Atherosclerosis and its manifestation in rheumatic diseases

3.1 Rheumatoid arthritis

RA is relatively the most common autoimmune disease with prevalence of 1%, which primarily affects joints and can also manifest by extra-articular involvement. The most frequent occurrence of RA is in middle-aged women. It can shorten the life expectancy by up to 2.5 years [89, 90]. In addition, there is up to three times higher mortality in RA patients compared to the general population [91]. CV involvement and complications, including asymptomatic heart failure or silent MI and sudden death, are the leading death causes in RA patients and occur in RA patients 1.5 times more often than in the general population [2, 92]. CV risk in RA is comparable to the risk in diabetes [93].

The underlying mechanism of increased CV mortality in RA is not completely understood [94]. The main cause of death in RA is ischemic heart disease (IHD), often asymptomatic and underdiagnosed [91, 95, 96]. Up to three times increased risk of IHD in RA patients with positivity of anti-cyclic citrullinated peptide (aCCP) antibodies and rheumatoid factor (RF) has been reported [69, 97].

In fact, RA itself can act as an independent risk factor for development of CVD [98]. The relation between an increase in the CV risk and the disease duration of RA patients is partly attributable to a higher prevalence of hypertension and smoking [99]. In RA, CV risk is also significantly related to traditional risk factors [100]. Smoking has a negative impact on the course of RA and stimulates the production of RF and aCCP nevertheless, the direct role in the increase of CV risk was not proved [98, 101].

Systemic inflammation accompanying the activity of RA significantly contributes to the atherogenesis and CV mortality [102]. The reduction of CV risk was observed during the DMARD therapy (namely HCQ, MTX, anti-TNFs). According to available studies and their meta-analysis, CV risk is most increased by CS therapy (up to 47%) and NSAIDs, in particular by coxibs (by 36%), and, on the contrary, is decreased by MTX (by 28%) or anti-TNF therapy (by about 30%) [72].

3.2 Ankylosing spondylitis

AS is a chronic inflammatory disease, which primarily affects the joints in the site of enthesis. It belongs to the group of diagnostic entity called spondyloarthropathies, which typically manifest in HLA-B27 positive patients. Similar to RA, AS can also manifest with extra-articular manifestations, such as gastrointestinal, ocular and cardiac involvement. The prevalence of AS in the population is about 0.1% (the overall prevalence of spondyloarthritis is around 1%) and, unlike most rheumatic diseases, occurs more frequently in men (up to three times) [103].

Similar to RA, an increased CV risk has been reported in AS patients [104, 105]. However, views on the close association of ATS and AS are divergent, in particular, due to the small evidence and conflicting results of studies [106]. Regarding the evidence on CV events in AS, the situation is similarly unsatisfactory and inconclusive [107–109]. Recently published meta-analysis has reported an increased risk of MI (RR = 1.6) and cerebrovascular events (RR = 1.5) compared to the general population [110].

There are several risk factors in AS, which participate in CV comorbidities. Since laboratory markers of inflammation are not elevated in many patients, CV risk is likely related to the risk profile of a typical patient with AS: a smoker with arterial hypertension and dyslipidemia, in whom low levels of HDL and TC accompany the disease activity [105, 110]. In addition, extra-articular cardiac manifestations of AS (e.g., conduction disorders, aortic valve insufficiency, left ventricular dysfunction) contribute to CV morbidity and mortality [105]. Levels of C-reactive protein (CRP), therapy with NSAIDs and work disability are considered significant predictive factors of CV mortality in AS [111, 112]. NSAIDs as the first-line therapy with the highest safety profile should be prescribed for the shortest time period possible [110]. On the other hand, anti-TNFs have a favorable effect on the endothelial function and a decrease of the CV risk [105, 113].

3.3 Psoriatic arthritis

PsA is a systemic inflammatory disease from the spondyloarthritis spectrum, associated with psoriasis [114]. The prevalence is 0.05–0.25% in the general population, but rises to 15–30% in patients with psoriasis [115]. The relative risk of CV involvement in psoriasis is reported to be 1.4, but the relative risk in PsA is less studied and the data are conflicting [116–119]. Meta-analysis demonstrated a 1.43 fold higher CV risk in PsA patients compared to the general population. The incidence of MI, cerebrovascular events and heart failure has been reported to be increased (1.68, 1.22 and 1.31, respectively) [120].

According to the current evidence, various manifestations of ATS in PsA have been described, from subclinical involvement to symptomatic manifestations [121–125]. PsA is considered to be an additional independent CV risk factor, as proved by findings of more severe subclinical ATS compared to the general population and the association of plaque development with the inflammatory activity of PsA [120].

PsA is typically associated with high prevalence of MetS, which is two or three times more common than in other rheumatic diseases and the general population [126]. During the active inflammatory phase, there are characteristic alterations of lipidogram with a decrease of HDL and LDL, which consequently rises in remission of the disease [9]. The suggested mechanism, which causes changes of HDL levels, is the uptake of apoA-1 in the tissue affected by inflammation: particles of HDL penetrate from the circulation due to increased endothelial permeability. The consequent decline of serum HDL concentrations increases the CV risk in PsA in a similar manner as in RA [127].

The presence of subclinical ATS and its correlation with inflammatory markers and the effect of immunosuppressive therapy are questionable [9, 128]. Anti-TFN therapy seems to have a beneficial effect on CV risk in PsA, as well as in AS [129].

3.4 Systemic lupus erythematosus

SLE is characterized by a wide spectrum of clinical manifestations and involvement of different organs. The prevalence is 0.03% in Caucasian population, while SLE affects predominantly women in reproductive years, in whom the clinically significant ATS is not usually found under normal circumstances [130]. Although the survival of SLE has significantly improved, thanks to new therapeutic options, it still remains 5–10 years shorter compared to the general population [131]. The rate of SLE-associated mortality has declined, but the rate of CV complications, which are considered to be the leading cause of mortality in SLE nowadays and are responsible for 30% of deaths, has risen [131]. The bimodal mortality pattern describes two peaks of mortality in SLE population: the first peak represents death early in the course of the disease related to the disease activity and infectious complications, and the second peak refers to late death from the CV manifestations [132].

The prevalence of traditional risk factors is higher in SLE compared to the general population [133]. In addition, SLE-related risk factors, including renal involvement, apply in CV morbidity. The presence of SLE itself increases the risk of heart failure up to three times [134]. The clinical manifestation of ATS in SLE is predicted particularly by higher age at the onset of SLE, presence of arterial hypertension and hypercholesterolemia. Among others, the cumulative dose and the duration of CS therapy, long duration of SLE, and activity of immune system including autoantibodies play significant role in ATS [2].

Due to their pathophysiologic mechanism both SLE and vasculitis predispose to the atherosclerotic involvement of coronary circulation [135]. Coronary artery disease affects 6–10% of SLE patients and the incidence is four to eight times higher than in the general population [136, 137].

Risk of heart failure in SLE significantly rises immediately after the first manifestation of the autoimmune disorder, mostly at a young age. The relative risk of heart failure is therefore most increased in young patients in the age between 20 and 30 years, and decreases with a higher age. However, the incidence of CV diseases and heart failure is continually increasing in positive correlation with the increasing age of patients [134]. SLE patients are at 5–10 times higher risk, and young SLE women at age around 40 years are even at 50 times higher risk of MI compared to the general population [138].

Concerning the risk of a stroke in SLE, the ischemic stroke is estimated to be two times, hemorrhagic stroke three times and subarachnoid hemorrhage four times more common in SLE than in the general population [139]. In case of a stroke, young patients are more threatened due to accelerated ATS during the high activity of inflammation. The relation between disease activity and the risk of a stroke was described also in other diseases. Immunosuppressive therapy and other comorbidities (e.g., vasculitis, antiphospholipid syndrome, arterial hypertension) take part in this increased risk, as well [139]. Accompanying factors such as antiphospholipid syndrome, Liebman-Sacks endocarditis and formation of immune complexes of antibodies with antigens predispose patients to thrombotic complications and ischemic stroke, while endothelial dysfunction and interrupted endothelial layer integrity can lead to hemorrhagic stroke. Subarachnoid hemorrhage in SLE probably results from intracerebral vasculitis and concurrent arterial hypertension [139].

Atherosclerotic plaques have been detected in 17–65% of SLE patients using ultrasound examination. The age seems to play a major role in prediction of atherosclerosis and its manifestations in SLE. Some experts suggest a role of consequences of the disease activity and side effects of therapy in older patients with SLE [2].

3.5 Systemic sclerosis

SSc belongs to orphan connective tissue diseases with the prevalence of 0.003–0.06%, and is less understood, concerning the CV risk. The key pathologies leading to CV involvement are vasculopathy, inflammation and tissue fibrosis, which can also affect the heart. In addition to pathognomic microvasculopathy, macrovascular involvement is getting more attention in the last years [45].

To date, the relative risk of CV diseases in SSc in not known. Survival of SSc patients is about 16–34 years shorter compared to the general population with about

3.5 times higher mortality [140]. Due to advances in therapy of scleroderma renal crisis (SRC) and pulmonary arterial hypertension (PAH), new causes of death have got to the front, and the prevalence of ATS in SSc has risen [141]. Cardiac causes account for a quarter of the overall mortality in SSc patients [142]. The prevalence of traditional CV risk does not seem to differ from the general population. SSc-associated factors, which participate in endothelial damage, include inflammation and ischemia-reperfusion injury caused by impaired vasodilation [45]. The level of inflammation in SSc is lower than in RA or SLE, which indicates lower rate of acceleration of ATS. Impaired vasodilation characteristic for both SSc and ATS precedes the clinical manifestation of SSc. It is accompanied by the mechanisms typical for both of these pathologies: imbalance between vasodilators (e.g., nitric oxide, NO) and vasoconstrictors (e.g., endothelin), defective angiogenesis caused by the increased expression of VEGF, the presence of AECA and others. The main clinical manifestations of microvascular impairment, Raynaud's phenomenon, PAH and SRC, probably predict macrovascular impairment in SSc [45].

Reports on the prevalence of ATS and its clinical manifestations in SSc differ in various studies. Among others, the reason is asymptomatic subclinical cardiac involvement. Increased risk of CV events is attributed both to ATS and the pathogenesis of SSc and its consequences (impaired microcirculation, myocardial fibrosis, arrhythmia, etc.), and last but not least, secondary deterioration of cardiac function due to renal vasculopathy, interstitial lung disease (ILD) and PAH [143].

The risk of MI is almost 2.5 times higher compared to the general population, while the impact of SSc itself outweighs the effect of hypertension or diabetes on the risk of MI. Ischemic injury of myocardium can be caused by occlusive vasculopathy and intermittent vasospasm (so-called myocardial Raynaud's phenomenon) [144].

It is not clear whether the prevalence of subclinical ATS in SSc is higher compared to the general population. Nussinovitch and Shoenfeld reported carotid involvement in more than 60% of SSc patients, where the findings were described to be more frequent and more severe than in a control group from the general population [143].

Cerebrovascular involvement in SSc patients is 1.3 times more common than in the general population. SSc as an independent risk factor increases the risk of ischemic stroke by up to 43%. There are several pathologic mechanisms in SSc playing a role in the manifestation of a stroke, including vasospasm of cerebral arteries corresponding to the Raynaud's phenomenon, which can manifest as a transient ischemic attack or a focal neurologic deficit [145].

3.6 Idiopathic inflammatory myopathies

IIM is a heterogeneous group of diseases, which primary affect the skeletal muscles as the common pathologic mechanism. The most prevalent subtypes are dermatomyositis (DM) and polymyositis (PM) [146, 147]. IIM belongs to orphan rheumatologic diseases and occurs in approximately 0.02% of population [148]. The mortality in IIM is almost four times higher than in the general population, with CV involvement as the leading cause [149]. The main pathology responsible for the cardiac involvement in IIM is myocarditis and accelerated ATS in coronary arteries [150]. Other mechanisms have not been sufficiently studied. Resulting structural alterations in myocardium can lead to disturbed function, arrhythmia and other, mostly asymptomatic, rarely fatal manifestations [151].

Data on cardiovascular disability in IIM are insufficient. Meta-analysis of studies in IIM reported 2.24 times higher CV risk compared to the general population [152]. With regard to the prevalence of MI in IIM, there are only limited data. A retrospective study by Rai et al. in more than 700 IIM patients described an increased risk of MI, but not of a stroke. The risk of MI has been increased in FM almost four times and in DM three times compared to the general population. Patients were most threatened by these complications during the first years after the onset of IIM [153].

Traditional risk factors in IIM are specifically related to the specific features of the disease, particularly muscle involvement resulting in impaired physical activity and CS therapy. The prevailing effect of CS in IIM, whether anti-inflammatory or pro-atherogenic, is not clear and has yet to be elucidated [152].

3.7 Primary Sjögren's syndrome

Primary Sjögren's syndrome is another relatively rare rheumatic disease with a prevalence of 0.06%. It is characterized by lymphocytic infiltration of exocrine glands (especially lacrimal and salivary) leading to dryness of the mucous membranes (sicca syndrome) and hyperactivity of B lymphocytes. pSS affects preferentially females at the age of 40–60 years [154].

The situation in terms of the CV risk in pSS is similarly unclear as in the above-mentioned rare systemic connective tissue diseases [155]. There is a lack of studies concerning the CV risk in pSS, moreover, the results are conflicting. CVD-associated mortality accounts for 30% of deaths. According to the recent meta-analysis including 14 studies in pSS, the CV risk is significantly increased compared to the general population: the relative risk of coronary artery disease is 1 34, cerebrovascular events 1.46, heart failure 2.54 and thromboembolism 1.78. This meta-analysis has not demonstrated a significantly increased risk of mortality due to CV causes (RR = 1.48) [155].

Similar results have been reported in a population study that also described higher prevalence of arterial hypertension and hypercholesterolemia in pSS patients, and, in addition, suggested pSS as an independent CV risk factor [156]. On the other hand, some studies did not confirm the increased CV risk in pSS [157, 158]. One study has reported subclinical atherosclerotic involvement in pSS patients detected by coronary flow reserve (CFR) and pulse wave velocity (PWV), while the echocardiography showed no pathology [159]. Impaired PWV is thus suggested as a marker of endothelial dysfunction even in patients with normal CFR [160].

Available data rather suggest higher CV risk in pSS patients compared to the general population, and the need of preventive screening and appropriate management, eventually including consultation and monitoring by a cardiologist [155].

4. Examination and estimation of the CV risk

Chronic inflammatory condition can skew the results of the examination, which have otherwise good reliability in the general population [3]. For example, ultrasound imaging of clinically insignificant atherosclerotic lesions or plaques cannot reveal the higher susceptibility to the progression and rupture of plaques in the inflammatory environment [5]. Several scoring systems were developed to facilitate the estimation of the CV risk in the general population. These scoring systems include particularly the traditional risk factors. The most used and widespread systems are Framingham Risk Score (FRS), Systemic Coronary Risk Evaluation (SCORE), QResearch Risk Score (QRISK2, or rather its updated version QRISK 3), Reynolds Risk Score and many others [161, 162]. FRS was the first developed scoring system and served as a default model for creating newer scoring systems. Nowadays, SCORE is probably the most used and widespread scoring system, especially in Europe [163]. Above-mentioned classic scoring systems underestimate the CV risk in rheumatic patients and therefore are not suitable for estimating the CV risk in these patients. A certain compromise was made by developing the Reynolds Risk Score by inclusion of CRP value as a marker of inflammation, and QRISK2 by inclusion the presence of RA as an independent risk factor [161]. Based on the recent EULAR recommendations for management of the CV risk in inflammatory arthropathies published in 2016, a modified SCORE system (mSCORE) should be used for evaluation of the CV risk in RA patients, which is calculated by multiplying the standard calculated value by a coefficient of 1.5 in all RA patients [58]. Despite this modification, mSCORE is not completely reliable in estimation of the CV risk, as was shown in studies describing findings of subclinical ATS in rheumatic patients classified in the low-risk category according to the mSCORE, and the evidence of higher tendency to formation of ATS plaques and instability of these plaques in RA. Due to these reasons, EULAR proposed simultaneous regular non-invasive examination by ultrasound of carotids and/or measuring the ankle-brachial index (ABI) for detection of subclinical ATS in asymptomatic patients in a low-risk category (SCORE 1–4%) [58, 82].

The CV risk should be assessed at least every 5 years in patients with low disease activity and should be reconsidered after major changes in therapy or progression of the disease [58, 59, 82]. In common practise, this assessment means regular examination of blood pressure and lipidogram during the outpatient control and in case of pathologic findings, early consultation by a preventive cardiologist and an adequate therapeutic intervention [62, 164].

5. Therapy

Preventive measures are the first-line therapy recommended in the general population to manage the CV risk. In rheumatic patients, these measures may be complicated due to a chronic disease. Therefore, the pharmacological treatment is needed [62, 82].

Metformin is recommended as the first line for the treatment of the MetS. It has a beneficial effect not only on improvement of insulin sensitivity, but also reduces the levels of LDL and TC and has a beneficial effect on the vascular function, as well as statins. Similar beneficial effect on glucose metabolism is related to administration of antimalarial drugs, which are often used in the treatment of SLE, pSS and also RA. HCQ exerts immunomodulatory and anti-inflammatory effect, and, in addition, induces an increase in insulin activity and serum levels of glucagon and improves the glucose tolerance. Moreover, HCQ reduces plasma glucose levels even in the general population and is therefore suitable as a part of MetS therapy [82]. Other drugs for glucose metabolism control include pioglitazone (a nuclear peroxisome proliferator-activated receptor-γ agonist), and liraglutide (glucagon-like peptide-1 analog), which has a beneficial effect in obese patients [13].

When managing and treating dyslipidemia, the recommended target levels of LDL (especially for RA) are lower than for the general population (LDL < 2.6 mmol/L; in individuals at higher risk, even <1.8 mmol/L). At the same time, preventive antiplatelet therapy should be considered [62]. Statins have been extensively discussed, especially in rheumatology. Via competitive inhibition of HMG-CoA (3-hydroxy-3-methyl-glutaryl-coenzym A) reductase, they inhibit the intermediate step in the synthesis of cholesterol. Despite the concerns of potential side effects as induction of immune-mediated necrotizing myopathy (IMNM), the use of statins in IIM patients does not seem to be more risky than in the general population [165]. Several studies demonstrated a beneficial potential of statins to reduce the CV risk via attenuation of the oxidative stress and improvement of endothelial function. Due to their anti-inflammatory potential, statins are preferentially recommended in the therapy of rheumatic patients according to the EULAR recommendations [62]. For example, atorvastatin, when administered to RA patients, not only reduces the levels of TC and LDL, but apparently also inhibits the inflammation activity [166]. This favorable effect was confirmed in TRACE-RA study [167]. Rosuvastatin exerts a similar beneficial effect in inflammatory joint diseases [168]. Another therapeutic option for dyslipidemia treatment is fenofibrate, which increases the HDL levels, and niacin [13].

Regarding the management of arterial hypertension, targeting the optimal blood pressure is more important than considering the type of drug used in therapy [58]. ACE inhibitors or blockers of AT1 receptor for angiotensin II exert a potential anti-inflammatory effect similar to statins, and therefore are preferentially recommended for treatment of arterial hypertension [62]. There is an exception in SSc patients. ACE inhibitors are recommended in the treatment of manifested SRC, but not as a prevention of SRC. Thus, other antihypertensive drugs should be prescribed (if SRC is not present), especially calcium channel blockers due to their beneficial effect on Raynaud's phenomenon [169].

Among other drugs with beneficial effect, vitamin D should not be forgotten. It was demonstrated that vitamin D acts as an immunomodulator and probably plays a protective role in the development of CV diseases, insulin resistance and obesity, and has anti-inflammatory effect and can potentially prevent from the development of MetS in RA patients. Also, probiotics are worth mentioning. Based on the results of studies showing that adverse changes of gut microbiome can induce autoimmune disorders, administration of probiotics may be profitable, as this could prevent the development of autoimmune disease or mitigate the consequences of already present pathological metabolic changes. However, further studies are needed to confirm these hypotheses [13].

Finally, the other side of this issue must not be forgotten, that is, adequate anti-inflammatory therapy of rheumatic diseases using DMARDs (especially MTX and TNF inhibitors in RA). Such therapy leads to mitigation of inflammatory activity and also improvement of quality of life and fitness of patients. Better fitness enables physical activity and thus facilitates the elimination of traditional risk factors and thereby reduces the CV risk [13].

6. Conclusion

Rheumatic patients are significantly more at risk of atherosclerosis and its complications than individuals from the general population. Traditional risk factors are in rheumatic patients more frequent. Moreover, these risk factors are often hard to manage by modification of life style. Nowadays, a wide range of therapeutic options is available for elimination of traditional risk factors and reduction of the cardiovascular risk. The appropriate anti-inflammatory therapy represents the golden standard. Despite the growing evidence on the cardiovascular risk in rheumatic patents, the adequate recommendations for management of these patients and early detection of a higher risk are still lacking. The task for the future is to create an examination algorithm to prevent underestimation and negligence of risk in rheumatic patients and also to extend the knowledge on the cardiovascular risk in rare rheumatic diseases.

Acknowledgements

This study was supported by AZV NV18-01-00161 A, MHCR 023728, and GAUK 312218.

Author details

Sabina Oreska and Michal Tomcik*
Department of Rheumatology, 1st Faculty of Medicine, Institute of Rheumatology,
Charles University, Prague, Czech Republic

*Address all correspondence to: michaltomcik@yahoo.com

IntechOpen

References

[1] Libby P, Lichtman AH, Hansson GK. Immune effector mechanisms implicated in atherosclerosis: From mice to humans. Immunity. 2013;**38**(6):1092-1104

[2] Sanjadi M et al. Atherosclerosis and autoimmunity: A growing relationship. International Journal of Rheumatic Diseases. 2018;**21**(5):908-921

[3] Catapano AL et al. ESC/EAS guidelines for the management of dyslipidaemias the task force for the management of dyslipidaemias of the European society of cardiology (ESC) and the European atherosclerosis society (EAS). Atherosclerosis. 2011;**217**(1):3-46

[4] Anderson KM et al. Cardiovascular disease risk profiles. American Heart Journal. 1991;**121**(1 Pt 2):293-298

[5] Kerekes G et al. Validated methods for assessment of subclinical atherosclerosis in rheumatology. Nature Reviews Rheumatology. 2012;**8**(4):224-234

[6] Castaneda S et al. Cardiovascular morbidity and associated risk factors in Spanish patients with chronic inflammatory rheumatic diseases attending rheumatology clinics: Baseline data of the CARMA project. Seminars in Arthritis and Rheumatism. 2015;**44**(6):618-626

[7] Amaya-Amaya J, Montoya-Sanchez L, Rojas-Villarraga A. Cardiovascular involvement in autoimmune diseases. BioMed Research International. 2014;**2014**:367359

[8] Libby P et al. Inflammation in atherosclerosis: From pathophysiology to practice. Journal of the American College of Cardiology. 2009;**54**(23):2129-2138

[9] Ramonda R et al. Atherosclerosis in psoriatic arthritis. Autoimmunity Reviews. 2011;**10**(12):773-778

[10] Sarmiento-Monroy JC et al. Cardiovascular disease in rheumatoid arthritis: A systematic literature review in latin america. Art. 2012;**2012**:371909

[11] Hess PL et al. The metabolic syndrome and risk of sudden cardiac death: The atherosclerosis risk in communities study. Journal of the American Heart Association. 2017;**6**(8):e006103

[12] Zmora N et al. The role of the immune system in metabolic health and disease. Cell Metabolism. 2017;**25**(3):506-521

[13] Medina G et al. Metabolic syndrome, autoimmunity and rheumatic diseases. Pharmacological Research. 2018;**133**:277-288

[14] Pfeiler S et al. IL-1 family cytokines in cardiovascular disease. Cytokine. 30 Nov 2017. pii: S1043-4666(17)30351-4. DOI: 10.1016/j.cyto.2017.11.009 [Epub ahead of print]

[15] van der Heijden T, Bot I, Kuiper J. The IL-12 cytokine family in cardiovascular diseases. Cytokine. 23 Oct 2017. pii: S1043-4666(17)30315-0. DOI: 10.1016/j.cyto.2017.10.010 [Epub ahead of print]

[16] Popovic-Kuzmanovic D et al. Increased activity of interleukin-23/interleukin-17 cytokine axis in primary antiphospholipid syndrome. Immunobiology. 2013;**218**(2):186-191

[17] Muniyappa R, Iantorno M, Quon MJ. An integrated view of insulin resistance and endothelial dysfunction. Endocrinology and Metabolism Clinics of North America. 2008;**37**(3):685-711, ix-x

[18] Shoelson SE, Lee J, Goldfine AB. Inflammation and insulin resistance. The Journal of Clinical Investigation. 2006;**116**(7):1793-1801

[19] Federico A et al. Gut microbiota, obesity and metabolic disorders. Minerva Gastroenterologica e Dietologica. 2017;**63**(4):337-344

[20] Abdollahi-Roodsaz S, Abramson SB, Scher JU. The metabolic role of the gut microbiota in health and rheumatic disease: Mechanisms and interventions. Nature Reviews Rheumatology. 2016;**12**(8):446-455

[21] Teh P, Zakhary B, Sandhu VK. The impact of obesity on SLE disease activity: Findings from the Southern California lupus registry (SCOLR). Clinical Rheumatology. 2019;**38**(2):597-600

[22] Nikiphorou E, Fragoulis GE. Inflammation, obesity and rheumatic disease: Common mechanistic links. A narrative review. Therapeutic Advances in Musculoskeletal Disease. 2018;**10**(8):157-167

[23] Riaz H et al. Association between obesity and cardiovascular outcomes: A systematic review and meta-analysis of mendelian randomization studies. JAMA Network Open. 2018;**1**(7):e183788

[24] Curtis JP et al. The obesity paradox: Body mass index and outcomes in patients with heart failure. Archives of Internal Medicine. 2005;**165**(1):55-61

[25] Cottam DR et al. The chronic inflammatory hypothesis for the morbidity associated with morbid obesity: Implications and effects of weight loss. Obesity Surgery. 2004;**14**(5):589-600

[26] Nishimura S et al. Adipose natural regulatory B cells negatively control adipose tissue inflammation. Cell Metabolism. 2013;**18**:759-766

[27] Osborn O, Olefsky JM. The cellular and signaling networks linking the immune system and metabolism in disease. Nature Medicine. 2012;**18**(3):363-374

[28] Rakhshandehroo M, Kalkhoven E, Boes M. Invariant natural killer T cells in adipose tissue: Novel regulators of immune-mediated metabolic disease. Cellular and Molecular Life Sciences. 2013;**70**(24):4711-4727

[29] Gremese E et al. Obesity as a risk and severity factor in rheumatic diseases (autoimmune chronic inflammatory diseases). Frontiers in Immunology. 2014;**5**:576

[30] Lumeng CN et al. Phenotypic switching of adipose tissue macrophages with obesity is generated by spatiotemporal differences in macrophage subtypes. Diabetes. 2008;**57**(12):3239-3246

[31] Versini M et al. Obesity in autoimmune diseases: Not a passive bystander. Autoimmunity Reviews. 2014;**13**(9):981-1000

[32] Sawicka K, Krasowska D. Adipokines in connective tissue diseases. Clinical and Experimental Rheumatology. 2016;**34**(6):1101-1112

[33] Feng W et al. Wendan decoction for dyslipidemia: Protocol for a systematic review and meta-analysis. Medicine. 2019;**98**(3):e14159

[34] Ganjali S et al. Monocyte-to-HDL-cholesterol ratio as a prognostic marker in cardiovascular diseases. Journal of Cellular Physiology. 2018;**233**(12):9237-9246

[35] Rosenson RS et al. Dysfunctional HDL and atherosclerotic cardiovascular disease. Nature Reviews Cardiology. 2016;**13**(1):48-60

[36] Rye KA et al. The metabolism and anti-atherogenic properties of

HDL. Journal of Lipid Research. 2009;**50**(Suppl):S195-S200

[37] Liao KP et al. Lipid and lipoprotein levels and trend in rheumatoid arthritis compared to the general population. Arthritis Care and Research. 2013;**65**(12):2046-2050

[38] Myasoedova E et al. Total cholesterol and LDL levels decrease before rheumatoid arthritis. Annals of the Rheumatic Diseases. 2010;**69**(7):1310-1314

[39] Crowson CS et al. Usefulness of risk scores to estimate the risk of cardiovascular disease in patients with rheumatoid arthritis. The American Journal of Cardiology. 2012;**110**(3):420-424

[40] Arts EE et al. Performance of four current risk algorithms in predicting cardiovascular events in patients with early rheumatoid arthritis. Annals of the Rheumatic Diseases. 2015;**74**(4):668-674

[41] Kawai VK et al. The ability of the 2013 American College of Cardiology/ American Heart Association cardiovascular risk score to identify rheumatoid arthritis patients with high coronary artery calcification scores. Arthritis & Rhematology. 2015;**67**(2):381-385

[42] Turiel M et al. Effects of long-term disease-modifying antirheumatic drugs on endothelial function in patients with early rheumatoid arthritis. Cardiovascular Therapeutics. 2010;**28**(5):e53-e64

[43] Kadayifci FZ, Karadag MG. The relationship of serum endocan levels and anti-TNF-alpha therapy in patients with ankylosing spondylitis. European Journal of Rheumatology. 2018;**5**(1):1-4

[44] Dhakal BP et al. Heart failure in systemic lupus erythematosus.

Trends in Cardiovascular Medicine. 2018;**28**(3):187-197

[45] Cannarile F et al. Cardiovascular disease in systemic sclerosis. Annals of Translational Medicine. 2015;**3**(1):8

[46] Shoenfeld Y, Sherer Y, Harats D. Artherosclerosis as an infectious, inflammatory and autoimmune disease. Trends in Immunology. 2001;**22**(6):293-295

[47] Prasad A et al. Predisposition to atherosclerosis by infections: Role of endothelial dysfunction. Circulation. 2002;**106**(2):184-190

[48] Zhou X et al. Transfer of CD4(+) T cells aggravates atherosclerosis in immunodeficient apolipoprotein E knockout mice. Circulation. 2000;**102**(24):2919-2922

[49] Wu R, Lefvert AK. Autoantibodies against oxidized low density lipoproteins (oxLDL): Characterization of antibody isotype, subclass, affinity and effect on the macrophage uptake of oxLDL. Clinical and Experimental Immunology. 1995;**102**(1):174-180

[50] Wu R et al. Antibodies against lysophosphatidylcholine and oxidized LDL in patients with SLE. Lupus. 1999;**8**(2):142-150

[51] Bergmark C et al. Patients with early-onset peripheral vascular disease have increased levels of autoantibodies against oxidized LDL. Arteriosclerosis, Thrombosis, and Vascular Biology. 1995;**15**(4):441-445

[52] Cinoku I et al. Autoantibodies to ox-LDL in Sjogren's syndrome: Are they atheroprotective? Clinical and Experimental Rheumatology. 2018;**36**(Suppl 112(3)):61-67

[53] George J et al. Immunolocalization of beta2-glycoprotein I (apolipoprotein H) to

human atherosclerotic plaques: Potential implications for lesion progression. Circulation. 1999;**99**(17):2227-2230

[54] Grainger DJ, Bethell HW. High titres of serum antinuclear antibodies, mostly directed against nucleolar antigens are associated with the presence of coronary atherosclerosis. Annals of the Rheumatic Diseases. 2002;**61**(2):110-114

[55] Liang KP et al. Autoantibodies and the risk of cardiovascular events. The Journal of Rheumatology. 2009;**36**(11):2462-2469

[56] Majka DS, Chang RW. Is preclinical autoimmunity benign?: The case of cardiovascular disease. Rheumatic Diseases Clinics of North America. 2014;**40**(4):659-668

[57] Husni ME. Comorbidities in psoriatic arthritis. Rheumatic Diseases Clinics of North America. 2015;**41**(4):677-698

[58] Agca R et al. EULAR recommendations for cardiovascular disease risk management in patients with rheumatoid arthritis and other forms of inflammatory joint disorders: 2015/2016 update. Annals of the Rheumatic Diseases. 2017;**76**(1):17-28

[59] Peters MJ et al. EULAR evidence-based recommendations for cardiovascular risk management in patients with rheumatoid arthritis and other forms of inflammatory arthritis. Annals of the Rheumatic Diseases. 2010;**69**(2):325-331

[60] Hallgren R, Berne C. Glucose intolerance in patients with chronic inflammatory diseases is normalized by glucocorticoids. Acta Medica Scandinavica. 1983;**213**(5):351-355

[61] Panoulas VF et al. Long-term exposure to medium-dose glucocorticoid therapy associates with hypertension in patients with rheumatoid arthritis. Rheumatology. 2008;**47**(1):72-75

[62] Nurmohamed MT, Heslinga M, Kitas GD. Cardiovascular comorbidity in rheumatic diseases. Nature Reviews Rheumatology. 2015;**11**(12):693-704

[63] Ruyssen-Witrand A et al. Cardiovascular risk induced by low-dose corticosteroids in rheumatoid arthritis: A systematic literature review. Joint, Bone, Spine. 2011;**78**(1):23-30

[64] Gargiulo P et al. Ischemic heart disease in systemic inflammatory diseases. An appraisal. International Journal of Cardiology. 2014;**170**(3):286-290

[65] Prasad M et al. Cardiorheumatology: Cardiac involvement in systemic rheumatic disease. Nature Reviews Cardiology. 2015;**12**(3):168-176

[66] Mercer E et al. Hydroxychloroquine improves insulin sensitivity in obese non-diabetic individuals. Arthritis Research & Therapy. 2012;**14**(3):R135

[67] Cairoli E et al. Hydroxychloroquine reduces low-density lipoprotein cholesterol levels in systemic lupus erythematosus: A longitudinal evaluation of the lipid-lowering effect. Lupus. 2012;**21**(11):1178-1182

[68] Floris A et al. Protective effects of hydroxychloroquine against accelerated atherosclerosis in systemic lupus erythematosus. Mediators of Inflammation. 2018;**2018**:3424136

[69] Myasoedova E et al. The influence of rheumatoid arthritis disease characteristics on heart failure. The Journal of Rheumatology. 2011;**38**(8):1601-1606

[70] Choi HK et al. Methotrexate and mortality in patients with rheumatoid

arthritis: A prospective study. Lancet. 2002;**359**(9313):1173-1177

[71] Wright K, Crowson CS, Gabriel SE. Cardiovascular comorbidity in rheumatic diseases: A focus on heart failure. Heart Failure Clinics. 2014;**10**(2):339-352

[72] Roubille C et al. The effects of tumour necrosis factor inhibitors, methotrexate, non-steroidal anti-inflammatory drugs and corticosteroids on cardiovascular events in rheumatoid arthritis, psoriasis and psoriatic arthritis: A systematic review and meta-analysis. Annals of the Rheumatic Diseases. 2015;**74**(3):480-489

[73] Ridker PM et al. Low-dose methotrexate for the prevention of atherosclerotic events. The New England Journal of Medicine. 2019;**380**(8):752-762

[74] Roubille C et al. Biologics and the cardiovascular system: A double-edged sword. Anti-Inflammatory & Anti-Allergy Agents in Medicinal Chemistry. 2013;**12**(1):68-82

[75] Micha R et al. Systematic review and meta-analysis of methotrexate use and risk of cardiovascular disease. The American Journal of Cardiology. 2011;**108**(9):1362-1370

[76] Westlake SL et al. Tumour necrosis factor antagonists and the risk of cardiovascular disease in patients with rheumatoid arthritis: A systematic literature review. Rheumatology. 2011;**50**(3):518-531

[77] Dixon WG et al. Reduction in the incidence of myocardial infarction in patients with rheumatoid arthritis who respond to anti-tumor necrosis factor alpha therapy: Results from the British society for rheumatology biologics register. Arthritis and Rheumatism. 2007;**56**(9):2905-2912

[78] Daien CI et al. Effect of TNF inhibitors on lipid profile in rheumatoid arthritis: A systematic review with meta-analysis. Annals of the Rheumatic Diseases. 2012;**71**(6):862-868

[79] Channual J, Wu JJ, Dann FJ. Effects of tumor necrosis factor-alpha blockade on metabolic syndrome components in psoriasis and psoriatic arthritis and additional lessons learned from rheumatoid arthritis. Dermatologic Therapy. 2009;**22**(1):61-73

[80] Antohe JL et al. Diabetes mellitus risk in rheumatoid arthritis: Reduced incidence with anti-tumor necrosis factor alpha therapy. Arthritis Care and Research. 2012;**64**(2):215-221

[81] Atzeni F et al. Investigating the potential side effects of anti-TNF therapy for rheumatoid arthritis: Cause for concern? Immunotherapy. 2015;**7**(4):353-361

[82] Martin-Martinez MA et al. Recommendations for the management of cardiovascular risk in patients with rheumatoid arthritis: Scientific evidence and expert opinion. Seminars in Arthritis and Rheumatism. 2014;**44**(1):1-8

[83] Interleukin-6 Receptor Mendelian Randomisation Analysis, C et al. The interleukin-6 receptor as a target for prevention of coronary heart disease: A mendelian randomisation analysis. Lancet. 2012;**379**(9822):1214-1224

[84] Kim SC et al. Cardiovascular safety of tocilizumab versus tumor necrosis factor inhibitors in patients with rheumatoid arthritis: A multi-database cohort study. Arthritis & Rhematology. 2017;**69**(6):1154-1164

[85] Kawashiri SY et al. Effects of the anti-interleukin-6 receptor antibody, tocilizumab, on serum lipid levels in patients with rheumatoid arthritis. Rheumatology International. 2011;**31**(4):451-456

[86] Pego-Reigosa JM et al. Long-term improvement of lipid profile in patients with refractory systemic lupus erythematosus treated with B-cell depletion therapy: A retrospective observational study. Rheumatology. 2010;**49**(4):691-696

[87] Kilickap S et al. Addition of rituximab to chop does not increase the risk of cardiotoxicity in patients with non-Hodgkin's lymphoma. Medical Oncology. 2008;**25**(4):437-442

[88] Ridker PM et al. Antiinflammatory therapy with canakinumab for atherosclerotic disease. The New England Journal of Medicine. 2017;**377**(12):1119-1131

[89] Kaneko Y, Takeuchi T. A paradigm shift in rheumatoid arthritis over the past decade. Internal Medicine. 2014;**53**(17):1895-1903

[90] Firestein GS. Evolving concepts of rheumatoid arthritis. Nature. 2003;**423**(6937):356-361

[91] Van Doornum S, McColl G, Wicks IP. Accelerated atherosclerosis: An extraarticular feature of rheumatoid arthritis? Arthritis and Rheumatism. 2002;**46**(4):862-873

[92] Mackey RH, Kuller LH, Moreland LW. Update on cardiovascular disease risk in patients with rheumatic diseases. Rheumatic Diseases Clinics of North America. 2018;**44**(3):475-487

[93] van Halm VP et al. Rheumatoid arthritis versus diabetes as a risk factor for cardiovascular disease: A cross-sectional study, the CARRE Investigation. Annals of the Rheumatic Diseases. 2009;**68**(9):1395-1400

[94] Solomon DH et al. Cardiovascular morbidity and mortality in women diagnosed with rheumatoid arthritis. Circulation. 2003;**107**(9):1303-1307

[95] Kaplan MJ, McCune WJ. New evidence for vascular disease in patients with early rheumatoid arthritis. Lancet. 2003;**361**(9363):1068-1069

[96] Zinger H, Sherer Y, Shoenfeld Y. Atherosclerosis in autoimmune rheumatic diseases-mechanisms and clinical findings. Clinical Reviews in Allergy and Immunology. 2009;**37**(1):20-28

[97] Lopez-Longo FJ et al. Association between anti-cyclic citrullinated peptide antibodies and ischemic heart disease in patients with rheumatoid arthritis. Arthritis and Rheumatism. 2009;**61**(4):419-424

[98] del Rincon ID et al. High incidence of cardiovascular events in a rheumatoid arthritis cohort not explained by traditional cardiac risk factors. Arthritis and Rheumatism. 2001;**44**(12):2737-2745

[99] Chung CP et al. Utility of the Framingham risk score to predict the presence of coronary atherosclerosis in patients with rheumatoid arthritis. Arthritis Research & Therapy. 2006;**8**(6):R186

[100] Boyer JF et al. Traditional cardiovascular risk factors in rheumatoid arthritis: A meta-analysis. Joint, Bone, Spine. 2011;**78**(2):179-183

[101] Shoenfeld Y et al. Accelerated atherosclerosis in autoimmune rheumatic diseases. Circulation. 2005;**112**(21):3337-3347

[102] Ridker PM. From C-reactive protein to interleukin-6 to interleukin-1: Moving upstream to identify novel targets for atheroprotection. Circulation Research. 2016;**118**(1):145-156

[103] Stolwijk C et al. Epidemiology of spondyloarthritis. Rheumatic Diseases Clinics of North America. 2012;**38**(3):441-476

[104] Papagoras C, Voulgari PV, Drosos AA. Atherosclerosis and cardiovascular disease in the spondyloarthritides, particularly ankylosing spondylitis and psoriatic arthritis. Clinical and Experimental Rheumatology. 2013;**31**(4):612-620

[105] Nurmohamed MT, van der Horst-Bruinsma I, Maksymowych WP. Cardiovascular and cerebrovascular diseases in ankylosing spondylitis: Current insights. Current Rheumatology Reports. 2012;**14**(5):415-421

[106] Peters MJ et al. Ankylosing spondylitis: A risk factor for myocardial infarction? Annals of the Rheumatic Diseases. 2010;**69**(3):579-581

[107] Mathieu S et al. Cardiovascular profile in ankylosing spondylitis: A systematic review and meta-analysis. Arthritis Care and Research. 2011;**63**(4):557-563

[108] Brophy S et al. No increased rate of acute myocardial infarction or stroke among patients with ankylosing spondylitis-a retrospective cohort study using routine data. Seminars in Arthritis and Rheumatism. 2012;**42**(2):140-145

[109] Chou CH et al. A nationwide population-based retrospective cohort study: Increased risk of acute coronary syndrome in patients with ankylosing spondylitis. Scandinavian Journal of Rheumatology. 2014;**43**(2):132-136

[110] Mathieu S, Pereira B, Soubrier M. Cardiovascular events in ankylosing spondylitis: An updated meta-analysis. Seminars in Arthritis and Rheumatism. 2015;**44**(5):551-555

[111] Bakland G, Gran JT, Nossent JC. Increased mortality in ankylosing spondylitis is related to disease activity. Annals of the Rheumatic Diseases. 2011;**70**(11):1921-1925

[112] Mok CC et al. Life expectancy, standardized mortality ratios, and causes of death in six rheumatic diseases in Hong Kong, China. Arthritis and Rheumatism. 2011;**63**(5):1182-1189

[113] Genre F et al. Anti-TNF-alpha therapy reduces endothelial cell activation in non-diabetic ankylosing spondylitis patients. Rheumatology International. 2015;**35**(12):2069-2078

[114] Braun J et al. 2010 update of the ASAS/EULAR recommendations for the management of ankylosing spondylitis. Annals of the Rheumatic Diseases. 2011;**70**(6):896-904

[115] Gladman DD et al. Psoriatic arthritis: Epidemiology, clinical features, course, and outcome. Annals of the Rheumatic Diseases. 2005;**64**(Suppl. 2):ii14-ii17

[116] Ahlehoff O et al. Psoriasis is associated with clinically significant cardiovascular risk: A Danish nationwide cohort study. Journal of Internal Medicine. 2011;**270**(2):147-157

[117] Kondratiouk S, Udaltsova N, Klatsky AL. Associations of psoriatic arthritis and cardiovascular conditions in a large population. The Permanente Journal. 2008;**12**(4):4-8

[118] Gladman DD et al. Cardiovascular morbidity in psoriatic arthritis. Annals of the Rheumatic Diseases. 2009;**68**(7):1131-1135

[119] Han C et al. Cardiovascular disease and risk factors in patients with rheumatoid arthritis, psoriatic arthritis, and ankylosing spondylitis. The Journal of Rheumatology. 2006;**33**(11):2167-2172

[120] Polachek A et al. Risk of cardiovascular morbidity in patients with psoriatic arthritis: A meta-analysis of observational studies. Arthritis Care & Research. 2017;**69**(1):67-74

[121] Eder L et al. Subclinical atherosclerosis in psoriatic arthritis: A case-control study. The Journal of Rheumatology. 2008;35(5):877-882

[122] Gonzalez-Juanatey C et al. High prevalence of subclinical atherosclerosis in psoriatic arthritis patients without clinically evident cardiovascular disease or classic atherosclerosis risk factors. Arthritis and Rheumatism. 2007;57(6):1074-1080

[123] Gonzalez-Juanatey C et al. Endothelial dysfunction in psoriatic arthritis patients without clinically evident cardiovascular disease or classic atherosclerosis risk factors. Arthritis and Rheumatism. 2007;57(2):287-293

[124] Tam LS et al. Subclinical carotid atherosclerosis in patients with psoriatic arthritis. Arthritis and Rheumatism. 2008;59(9):1322-1331

[125] Rose S et al. Psoriatic arthritis and sacroiliitis are associated with increased vascular inflammation by 18-fluorodeoxyglucose positron emission tomography computed tomography: Baseline report from the psoriasis atherosclerosis and cardiometabolic disease initiative. Arthritis Research & Therapy. 2014;16(4):R161

[126] Mok CC et al. Prevalence of atherosclerotic risk factors and the metabolic syndrome in patients with chronic inflammatory arthritis. Arthritis Care and Research. 2011;63(2):195-202

[127] Oliviero F et al. Apolipoprotein A-I and cholesterol in synovial fluid of patients with rheumatoid arthritis, psoriatic arthritis and osteoarthritis. Clinical and Experimental Rheumatology. 2009;27(1):79-83

[128] Kimhi O et al. Prevalence and risk factors of atherosclerosis in patients with psoriatic arthritis. Seminars in Arthritis and Rheumatism. 2007;36(4):203-209

[129] Angel K et al. Tumor necrosis factor-alpha antagonists improve aortic stiffness in patients with inflammatory arthropathies: A controlled study. Hypertension. 2010;55(2):333-338

[130] Cervera R et al. Morbidity and mortality in systemic lupus erythematosus during a 10-year period: A comparison of early and late manifestations in a cohort of 1,000 patients. Medicine. 2003;82(5):299-308

[131] Wigren M, Nilsson J, Kaplan MJ. Pathogenic immunity in systemic lupus erythematosus and atherosclerosis: Common mechanisms and possible targets for intervention. Journal of Internal Medicine. 2015;278(5):494-506

[132] Urowitz MB et al. The bimodal mortality pattern of systemic lupus erythematosus. The American Journal of Medicine. 1976;60(2):221-225

[133] Petri M et al. Coronary artery disease risk factors in the Johns Hopkins lupus cohort: Prevalence, recognition by patients, and preventive practices. Medicine. 1992;71(5):291-302

[134] Kim CH et al. Incidence and risk of heart failure in systemic lupus erythematosus. Heart. 2017;103(3):227-233

[135] Mason JC, Libby P. Cardiovascular disease in patients with chronic inflammation: Mechanisms underlying premature cardiovascular events in rheumatologic conditions. European Heart Journal. 2015;36(8):482-489c

[136] Petri M et al. Risk factors for coronary artery disease in patients with systemic lupus erythematosus. The American Journal of Medicine. 1992;93(5):513-519

[137] Manzi S et al. Age-specific incidence rates of myocardial infarction

and angina in women with systemic lupus erythematosus: Comparison with the Framingham study. American Journal of Epidemiology. 1997;**145**(5):408-415

[138] Schoenfeld SR, Kasturi S, Costenbader KH. The epidemiology of atherosclerotic cardiovascular disease among patients with SLE: A systematic review. Seminars in Arthritis and Rheumatism. 2013;**43**(1):77-95

[139] Holmqvist M et al. Stroke in systemic lupus erythematosus: A meta-analysis of population-based cohort studies. RMD Open. 2015;**1**(1):e000168

[140] Psarras A et al. A critical view on cardiovascular risk in systemic sclerosis. Rheumatology International. 2017;**37**(1):85-95

[141] Soriano A, Afeltra A, Shoenfeld Y. Is atherosclerosis accelerated in systemic sclerosis? Novel insights. Current Opinion in Rheumatology. 2014;**26**(6):653-657

[142] Rubio-Rivas M et al. Mortality and survival in systemic sclerosis: Systematic review and meta-analysis. Seminars in Arthritis and Rheumatism. 2014;**44**(2):208-219

[143] Nussinovitch U, Shoenfeld Y. Atherosclerosis and macrovascular involvement in systemic sclerosis: Myth or reality. Autoimmunity Reviews. 2011;**10**(5):259-266

[144] Man A et al. The risk of cardiovascular disease in systemic sclerosis: A population-based cohort study. Annals of the Rheumatic Diseases. 2013;**72**(7):1188-1193

[145] Chu SY et al. Increased risk of acute myocardial infarction in systemic sclerosis: A nationwide population-based study. The American Journal of Medicine. 2013;**126**(11):982-988

[146] Bohan A, Peter JB. Polymyositis and dermatomyositis (first of two parts). The New England Journal of Medicine. 1975;**292**(7):344-347

[147] Bohan A, Peter JB. Polymyositis and dermatomyositis (second of two parts). The New England Journal of Medicine. 1975;**292**(8):403-407

[148] Findlay AR, Goyal NA, Mozaffar T. An overview of polymyositis and dermatomyositis. Muscle & Nerve. 2015;**51**(5):638-656

[149] Dobloug GC et al. Mortality in idiopathic inflammatory myopathy: Results from a Swedish nationwide population-based cohort study. Annals of the Rheumatic Diseases. 2018;**77**(1):40-47

[150] Schwartz T et al. Cardiac involvement in adult and juvenile idiopathic inflammatory myopathies. RMD Open. 2016;**2**(2):e000291

[151] Diederichsen LP. Cardiovascular involvement in myositis. Current Opinion in Rheumatology. 2017;**29**(6):598-603

[152] Ungprasert P et al. Risk of coronary artery disease in patients with idiopathic inflammatory myopathies: A systematic review and meta-analysis of observational studies. Seminars in Arthritis and Rheumatism. 2014;**44**(1):63-67

[153] Rai SK et al. Risk of myocardial infarction and ischaemic stroke in adults with polymyositis and dermatomyositis: A general population-based study. Rheumatology. 2016;**55**(3):461-469

[154] Qin B et al. Epidemiology of primary Sjogren's syndrome: A systematic review and meta-analysis. Annals of the Rheumatic Diseases. 2015;**74**(11):1983-1989

[155] Beltai A et al. Cardiovascular morbidity and mortality in primary Sjogren syndrome: A systematic review and meta-analysis. Arthritis Care and Research (Hoboken). 20 Dec 2018. DOI: 10.1002/acr.23821 [Epub ahead of print]

[156] Bartoloni E et al. Cardiovascular disease risk burden in primary Sjogren's syndrome: Results of a population-based multicentre cohort study. Journal of Internal Medicine. 2015;**278**(2):185-192

[157] Chiang CH et al. Primary Sjogren's syndrome and the risk of acute myocardial infarction: A Nationwide study. Acta Cardiologica Sinica. 2013;**29**(2):124-131

[158] Chiang CH et al. Primary Sjogren's syndrome and risk of ischemic stroke: A nationwide study. Clinical Rheumatology. 2014;**33**(7):931-937

[159] Atzeni F et al. Can speckle tracking echocardiography detect subclinical left ventricular dysfunction in patients with primary Sjogren's syndrome? Clinical and Experimental Rheumatology. 2017;**35**(1):173

[160] Atzeni F et al. New parameters for identifying subclinical atherosclerosis in patients with primary Sjogren's syndrome: A pilot study. Clinical and Experimental Rheumatology. 2014;**32**(3):361-368

[161] Payne RA. Cardiovascular risk. British Journal of Clinical Pharmacology. 2012;**74**(3):396-410

[162] Hippisley-Cox J, Coupland C, Brindle P. Development and validation of QRISK3 risk prediction algorithms to estimate future risk of cardiovascular disease: Prospective cohort study. BMJ. 2017;**357**:j2099

[163] Conroy RM et al. Estimation of ten-year risk of fatal cardiovascular disease in Europe: The SCORE project. European Heart Journal. 2003;**24**(11):987-1003

[164] Piepoli MF et al. European Guidelines on cardiovascular disease prevention in clinical practice: The sixth joint task force of the european society of cardiology and other societies on cardiovascular disease prevention in clinical practice (constituted by representatives of 10 societies and by invited experts) developed with the special contribution of the European association for cardiovascular prevention & rehabilitation (EACPR). European Heart Journal. 2016;**2016, 37**(29):2315-2381

[165] Charles-Schoeman C et al. Treatment of dyslipidemia in idiopathic inflammatory myositis: Results of the International Myositis Assessment and Clinical Studies Group survey. Clinical Rheumatology. 2012;**31**:1163-1168, 1168

[166] McCarey DW et al. Trial of atorvastatin in rheumatoid arthritis (TARA): Double-blind, randomised placebo-controlled trial. Lancet. 2004;**363**(9426):2015-2021

[167] Kitas GD et al. Trial of atorvastatin for the primary prevention of cardiovascular events in patients with rheumatoid arthritis (TRACE RA): A multicenter, randomized, placebo controlled trial. Arthritis & Rheumatology. 15 Apr 2019. pp. 1-13. DOI: 10.1002/art.40892 [Epub ahead of print]

[168] Rollefstad S et al. Rosuvastatin-induced carotid plaque regression in patients with inflammatory joint diseases: The rosuvastatin in rheumatoid arthritis, ankylosing spondylitis and other inflammatory joint diseases study. Arthritis & Rheumatology. 2015;**67**(7):1718-1728

[169] Kowal-Bielecka O et al. Update of EULAR recommendations for the treatment of systemic sclerosis. Annals of the Rheumatic Diseases. 2017;**76**(8):1327-1339

Chapter 5

Atherosclerosis: A Journey around the Terminology

Oladimeji Adebayo and Abiodun Moshood Adeoye

Abstract

The term atherosclerosis underwent a tedious pathway to arrive at its current status and interpretation. Furthermore, terms such as atherosclerosis, arteriosclerosis and arteriolosclerosis appear similar and are misused interchangeably. This chapter highlighted the various terminologies linked with atherosclerosis. This chapter highlighted how the terminology of atherosclerosis evolved and, also, the various classifications, e.g., atherosclerosis, Monckeberg calcific sclerosis and arteriolosclerosis, and gave mention to the differences among them.

Keywords: atherosclerosis, arteriosclerosis, arteriolosclerosis

1. Introduction

The understanding of atherosclerosis evolved uniquely in terms of terminology, aetiology, structural features or pathophysiology over the last 300 years [1]. Furthermore, the three terms, atherosclerosis, arteriosclerosis and arteriolosclerosis, with lethal implications and similar terminologies affecting the arterial vessels, however, can easily be confused or just used interchangeably indiscriminately [1–5]. There is evidence in the literature that these terms are mistakenly interchanged [3, 4, 6]. This confusion was not helped by the key stakeholders like the pathologists and clinicians who over the years failed to reach a consensus to delineate them [7].

A remarkable example of such confusion is that emanating from the American Heart Association (AHA) who publishes journals titled *Arteriosclerosis, Thrombosis, and Vascular Biology* and *Hypertension*. While the *Arteriosclerosis, Thrombosis, and Vascular Biology* journal publishes mainly articles related to the experimental, clinical and epidemiological facets of atherosclerosis, the *Hypertension* journal has a prominent section on "arteriosclerosis" [6].

Interestingly the confusion around the nomenclature appears to be age-long. Hueper, WC's writing in the *Archives of Pathology and Laboratory Medicine* in 1945 titled "Arteriosclerosis" suggests the term atherosclerosis was extensively used concerning the pathology related to cholesterol metabolism [8]. Rabson a medical doctor while writing a letter to the editor of the American College of Clinical Pathology expressed his alarm at the confusion of the degenerative disease [8, 9]. This alarm was stemmed from the observation of an article titled arteriosclerosis, but the article did not use any of such nomenclature rather than atherosclerosis [9].

As recent as 1995, the AHA Report from the Committee on Vascular Lesions of the Council Arteriosclerosis interchanged arteriosclerosis and atherosclerosis [11].

Not that there are no prominent attempts to delineate these terms, especially for arteriosclerosis and atherosclerosis. As far back as 1963, George Pickering, one of the fathers of modern cardiology, highlighted the similar confusion between arteriosclerosis and atherosclerosis in his lecture at The University of Alabama, published in the article "Arteriosclerosis and Atherosclerosis: The Need for Clear Thinking" which stated the definition in clear terms [6, 7]. He believed the confusion might be as a result of affectation of the arterial system by the two entities although they affect different arterial sizes. He, however, delineated them by defining atherosclerosis as *a complex inflammatory process associated with the presence of oxidized low-density lipoprotein (LDL) cholesterol in the intima and media of the arterial wall* and arteriosclerosis as the *functional depletion of large artery elasticity* [6].

Also, notable observation is that arteriosclerosis [10] serves two functions, an overarching term for other sub-terms and merely a term that can be inter-used with atherosclerosis [2, 11]. Besides, there is poor agreement on the terms related to atherosclerosis.

Also, over the years, other terms such as Mönckeberg medial calcific sclerosis (MCS) and arteriolosclerosis gained popularity [1]. There was a feeble attempt for clear terms and classification as related to atherosclerosis.

The chapter will also highlight recommendations on possible reclassification based on gross and histopathologic features, among others. In summary, the chapter will extensively discuss the key terms related to arteriosclerosis and the historical evolution of these terms and highlight recommendations on possible reclassification as having been previously recommended and published.

2. Arteriosclerosis

Arteriosclerosis is derived from the Greek word arteria, meaning artery, and sclerosis, meaning hardening, and "osis" is a Greek suffix that means a diseased condition [14]. Much literature appears to refer to arteriosclerosis as the overarching term that includes three different lesions, atherosclerosis, arteriolosclerosis and Mönckeberg medial calcific sclerosis (**Figure 1**) [2, 12]. The three lesions are underpinned by the resultant hardening and thickening of the arterial wall [2]. However there appears not to be any consensus document by any significant cardiovascular or pathology organization on such division rather than such classification emanated from classic textbooks of pathology [1]. Many articles also carry this classification [13].

It, however, appears that the term is also used to describe the functional diminution of large artery elasticity marked by pulse wave velocity [14]. It, however, brings to fore another dimension of intermix with atherosclerosis.

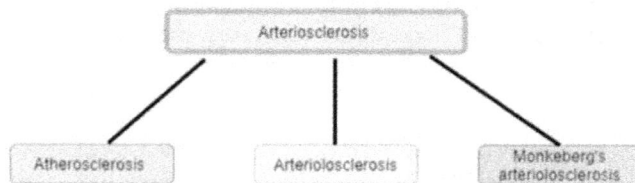

Figure 1.
The classification of arteriosclerosis.

3. Atherosclerosis

Atherosclerosis is derived from the Greek word "athero", meaning gruel or paste, and sclerosis, meaning hardening, and "osis" is a Greek suffix that describes a diseased condition [15]. It merely is the hardening of an artery precisely due to an atheromatous plaque. Atherosclerotic lesions otherwise called atheromata are asymmetric focal

Year	Milestones
1575	Fallopius wrote about "a degeneration of arteries into bone," and anatomists of that era commonly mentioned ossified arteries [2]
1740	Johann Friedrich Crell described this as the hardening of the vessels instead of bony arteries [17]
1755	von Haller described this hardening as thickening as "atheroma" [1, 37, 38]
1833	Frenchman Jean Frederic Martin Lobstein first used the term "arteriosclerosis" to describe calcified arterial lesions [1]
1868	George Johnson limited the term arteriosclerosis to "noncalcified, non-atheromatous stiffening of small vessels" [2]
1881	Jean Frederic Martin Lobstein first used the term arteriosclerosis in the second volume of his book titled *Traité d'Anatomie Pathologique* [17, 39]
1903	Mönckeberg arteriosclerosis was first described and named after Johann Georg Mönckeberg using details from 130 patients. It was also called "Mönckeberg media sclerosis" or "Mönckeberg media calcinosis" [38, 40]
1904	Félix Marchand introduced the term "atherosclerosis" and suggested it is responsible for obstructive processes in the arteries [2, 33, 41]
1908	A.I. Ignatowski demonstrated that rabbits experimentally develop atherosclerosis by feeding on cholesterol-rich food of egg and meat [33, 34]
1910	Adolf Windaus demonstrated that atheromatous plaque has a concentration of cholesterol [33, 42]
1914	Anitschkow described the role of cholesterol accumulation in the development of atherosclerosis [35]
2012	Faber differentiated calcification in the coronary arteries which are atherosclerotic in origin from Mönckeberg sclerosis [4]
1913	Nikolai N. Anichkov showed that cholesterol alone caused the atheromatous changes in the vascular wall [33, 43]
1954	Rabson SM noted that arteriosclerosis lacked specificity, uniformity and consistency. He suggested how the term would be used [2]
1961	Sir George Pickering, one of the fathers of modern cardiology in his lecture at the fourth Tinsley Randolph Harrison lecture at The University of Alabama, clearly differentiated arteriosclerosis and atherosclerosis
1965	Eggen and other workers demonstrated atherosclerotic coronary artery calcification [4]
1971	Russell Ross and Seymour J. Klebanoff using electron microscopy demonstrated that the atherosclerosis lesions are characterized by an accumulation of smooth muscle cells associated with abundant connective tissue matrix [44]
1972	Ross and colleagues showed that vascular smooth muscle cells proliferate and synthesize and secrete all three major constituents of connective tissue: collagen, elastic fibre microfibrils and elastin
1975	Watanabe heritable hyperlipidaemic rabbits were discovered and subsequently used in most experimental settings for lipid disorder and atherosclerosis [45]
1985	Brown and Goldstein discovered the role of low-density lipoprotein (LDL) receptors which won them the 1985 Nobel Prize
1992	The AHA started to release a series to define the intima of human arteries and its atherosclerosis-prone regions
1995	The AHA published the last of report classifying atherosclerosis using histological composition and structure [11]

Table 1.
Key milestone which refined the term atherosclerosis and related terms.

Atherosclerosis [18]	Arteriolosclerosis	Mönckeberg arteriosclerosis
Dyslipidaemia		Dyslipidaemia
Hypertension	Hypertension	
Diabetes mellitus	Diabetes mellitus	Diabetes mellitus
Genetic risk factors	Genetic risk factors such as ABCC9 gene variant	Genetic diseases such as Keutel syndrome
Inflammation		Chronic inflammatory disease such as systemic lupus erythematosus, etc.
Ageing	Ageing	Ageing
		Disturbances of calcium metabolism
Obesity		
Family history of early heart disease or coronary heart disease		
	Chronic kidney disease	Chronic kidney disease
Smoking and other tobacco use		
High level of CRP		
Alcohol		
Sleep apnoea		
Sedentary lifestyle		
Fibrinogen level		
Type A personality type		
Air pollution		
	Blood-brain barrier dysfunctions	

Table 2.
The risk factors associated with atherosclerosis, arteriolosclerosis and Mönckeberg's arteriosclerosis.

	Atherosclerosis	Arteriolosclerosis	Mönckeberg arteriosclerosis
Key processes	Lipid accumulation	Protein accumulation and fibromuscular proliferation of the intima	Calcium deposition
Type of process	Pathologic	Pathologic	Physiology and pathologic
Vessels affected	Large and medium arteries	Concentric media thickening of muscular arteries	
Part of the vessel affected	Intima and underlying smooth muscle	Media	Internal elastic lamina
Pathomorphological	Plaque-forming degenerative changes of the large elastic arteries such as the aorta	Thickening of the vessel walls that narrows the lumen	Patchy calcification of the intima
Effect on vessel dimension	Decrease	Decrease	Nil
Calcification	++		+++

Table 3.
Some key differences in atherosclerosis, arteriolosclerosis and Mönckeberg arteriosclerosis.

thickenings of the intima which is the innermost layer of the artery [16]. While arteriosclerosis is a chronic pathological disease concept which refers to arterial lesions characterized by intimal thickening, stiffening and remodelling of the arterial walls [2]. Atherosclerosis is a generic term used to describe a general term describing a hardening of medium or large arteries [1, 2]. It is also referred to as atherosclerotic vascular disease.

The atheroma principally blocks large- and medium-sized elastic and muscular arteries leading to ischemia in the heart, brain or extremities, thereby causing infarction [17]. The most critical risk factor for atherosclerosis is dyslipidaemia due to high plasma concentrations of cholesterol, especially low-density lipoprotein (LDL) cholesterol or high-density lipoprotein. While dyslipidaemia is a key risk factor, it can be found at age (**Tables 1–3**) [17]. The critical step in atherosclerosis formation includes (i) fatty streak formation, (ii) atheroma formation and (iii) atherosclerotic plaque formation [18].

4. Arteriolosclerosis

Arteriolosclerosis is simply the hardening and loss of the elasticity of the small arteries and arterioles due to the progressive increase in the elastic and muscular components of the wall of those vessels. It is simply the small vessel disease and principally affects the brain and the kidneys [19, 20]. In the brain, it is associated with the lacunar infarcts, vascular cognitive impairment and diffuse white matter lesions [19]. The key predisposing factors include hypertension, ageing, ABCC9 gene variant, diabetes mellitus and blood-brain barrier dysfunctions (**Tables 2** and **3**) [21]. The sub-types include hyaline arteriolosclerosis and hyperplastic arteriolosclerosis.

5. Mönckeberg medial calcific sclerosis (MCS)

Monckeberg medial calcific sclerosis (MCS), Mönckeberg arteriosclerosis, or Mönckeberg sclerosis is a degenerative and noninflammatory disease in which the media of medium-sized and small muscular arteries becomes calcified independent of atherosclerosis [22]. It is also considered as atherosclerotic medial calcification [4]. It is a ringlike calcification of the vascular media of small- to medium-sized vessels without associated intimal thickening [22, 23]. It is a form of arteriosclerosis or vessel hardening, where calcium deposits are in the muscular middle layer of the walls of arteries (the tunica media). It usually causes damage to the kidney and heart.

Mönckeberg arteriosclerosis is commonly mixed up with calciphylaxis and probably is the most controversial type of arteriosclerosis [4, 24].

6. Historical background of atherosclerosis

Atherosclerosis or other related nomenclatures are not new disease entities (**Tables 2** and **3**). There was, however, some emerging insight into what was later termed as atherosclerosis. Hippocrates (469–377 BC), the father of modern medicine, described the sudden cardiac death, while approximately 300 BC, Erasistratus described the typical claudication intermittent symptoms of peripheral arterial disease [25].

Egyptian mummies were noted to have evidence of atherosclerosis; although this was not yet named atherosclerosis [8, 26–28]. In the earlier times, due to the lack of sophisticated equipment to help the understanding, degenerative and nondegenerative arteriopathy was also lumped together and poorly delineated. However, the understanding of atherosclerosis increased exponentially in the last seven decades, even though it was earlier thought to be a mere accomplishment of ageing and dodged for many years with controversies surrounding its link with cholesterol [27].

Albrecht von Haller, a Swiss biologist and the father of experimental physiology, used the Latin term "atheroma," in 1755, to describe the plaque deposited on the innermost layer of systemic artery walls [29]. However it appears that Celsius may have used the same word about 2000 years ago while describing a fatty tumour [30].

In 1575, Fallopius wrote about "a degeneration of arteries into bone" suggestive of the presence of calcified atherosclerotic lesions in the arteries. Furthermore, ossified arteries were commonly mentioned by anatomists of that era [2]. By the eighteenth century, it was apparent that some progress has been made in understanding albeit rudimentary on what we call atherosclerosis today. For example, in 1799, Parry suggested the relationship between coronary lesions and the symptoms of angina pectoris [25].

Also, in 1815, J. Hodgson defined the fatty arterial degeneration as atheromatosis [30].

Frenchman Jean Frederic Martin Lobstein first used the term "arteriosclerosis" to describe calcified arterial lesions in his main body of work, a four-volume work on pathological anatomy written in French titled *Traité d'Anatomie Pathologique (Treatise on Pathological Anatomy)*, based upon his vast personal experience [1, 25]. The work was unfinished at the time of his death in 1835.

The first mention of nondegenerative arteriopathy in the textbook was by Maurice Raynaud's in *De l'Asphyxie Locale et de la Gangrene Symetrique des Extremites* (1852) and Leo Buerger's "Thromboangiitis obliterans" [31]. While in 1879, more than 80 years later, Potain interpreted the relationship Parry found to arise from myocardial ischemia [25].

From 1900 onwards, the most significant progress in the understanding of atherosclerosis was made. At the beginning of the twentieth century, Aschoff introduced atherosis and atherosclerosis to describe morphologically different intimal lipid deposits of children and adults as early and late stages, respectively [32].

By 1904, Félix Marchand suggested that "atherosclerosis" should be better instead of "atheroma" as earlier described by Haller [29]. He had combined two Greek root words: *athéré, which* meant gruel or porridge, and *sclerosis*, which signifies hardening [29]. He did not only gave a nomenclature currently in use, but he also did justice to the pathologic process involving the association of fatty degeneration and vessel stiffening. He believed that atherosclerosis was responsible for almost all obstructive processes in the arteries [33]. In 1910, Adolf Windaus demonstrated that aortic "atheromatous lesions" contained six times as much as free cholesterol and 20-fold of esterified cholesterol compared to normal aortic wall [27, 33]. A.I. Ignatowski demonstrated that rabbits experimentally develop atherosclerosis by feeding on cholesterol-rich food of egg and meat [33, 34].

In 1914, Anitschkow, influenced by Ignatowski's work, gave the first description of the role of cholesterol accumulation in the development of atherosclerosis while emphasizing the cardinal role of cholesterol in atheromatous changes in the vascular wall [35]. He had used a cholesterol-fed rabbit model while working at the Military Medical Academy in St. Petersburg to demonstrate that the extent of atherosclerosis was proportional to the absolute amount of and length of exposure to high blood cholesterol [27, 35]. His discovery was a defining moment in the study of this disease entity, although not without scepticism. While the rabbit model develops atherosclerosis after being fed high amounts of meat, eggs and milk, the dog and rat model did not [33]. This finding by later workers almost torpedoed this discovery attributable to Anitschkow [27]. It was also a blow to the lipid hypothesis due to these later species relative resistance to diet-induced hypercholesterolemia. Other factors that may have eroded the most unequivocal link of cholesterol and atherosclerosis as enunciated by Anitschkow was the prevailing senescence hypothesis as a plausible reason for the development of atherosclerosis when he made the discovery [27]. Anitschkow also first described the *cholester-inesterphagozyten*, which today commonly is known as foam cells, derived from macrophages [25, 35].

The discussion of lipid hypothesis generally in the first 50 years of the twentieth century was also dodged with controversy, particularly the role of high blood cholesterol levels to the causal relationship of atherosclerosis and coronary heart disease, and that atherosclerosis was a reward of ageing as espoused by senescence hypothesis [27, 36].

With the improvement in morphological, immunohistological and molecular methods and advanced investigative techniques, LDL receptor and its roles in the development of atherosclerosis were discovered by Brown and Goldstein [25]. By 1958, there was enough information to make classification of atherosclerosis by the World Health Organization and described the sequences as a fatty streak, atheroma, fibrous plaque and complicated lesions [32]. The American Heart Association (AHA) starting from 1992 proposed a new morphological classification based on eight lesion types designated by Roman numerals which indicate the usual sequence of lesion progression [32].

Jian-Jun Li and Chun-Hong Fang's writing in *Medical Hypotheses* journal suggests that atheroscleritis is a more rational term for atherosclerosis [29].

We now know the pathological processes that underpin atherosclerosis, which entails (1) endothelial injury, (2) intimal cholesterol accumulation and monocyte invasion with subsequent foam cell formation, (3) migration and proliferation of smooth muscle cells with expression of extracellular matrix, (4) local thrombus formation with secondary organization, (5) calcification and/or plaque rupture and (6) final occlusion due to plaque rupture/thrombus formation [25].

7. Challenges with terms

Gregory et al. pointed out the difficulty with terms which they notice: (i) it has an inconsistent naming convention, (ii) it fails to use terms that accurately describe the lesions, (iii) significant sclerotic arterial lesions are absent from the classification, and (iv) interchangeability of arteriosclerosis and atherosclerosis [2]:

1. **Naming convention.** The three authors noticed that the arteriosclerosis, atherosclerosis and Mönckeberg medial sclerosis are defined by their gross and histopathologic attributes while arteriolosclerosis was defined by vessel dimension [2]. Furthermore, "arteriolo" is a descriptive pathologic term.

2. **Description of lesion.** This term poorly describes the terms [2]. The Mönckeberg medial sclerosis as described by Mönckeberg, ironically, may not be described, and the lesion may involve the arterial intima rather than the arterial media [2]. Furthermore, arteriolosclerosis, which is a hardening of the vessel, does not describe the lesion since the process involves both protein accumulation and fibromuscular proliferation of the intima [1].

3. **Absence of crucial lesion from the classifications.** Restenosis lesions after balloon angioplasty and stenting, transplant arteriopathy, intimal nonatherosclerotic proliferative lesions in arterial vessels larger than arterioles, and a variety of disorders associated with vascular calcification are not yet included in the current classification.

Although Gregory et al. highlighted the problems with terms, they retained the classifications which do not have all the necessary inclusion [2]. They suggested atherosclerosis, primary arterial calcification, fibromuscular intimal hyperplasia, hyalinosis, and miscellaneous categories which include amyloidosis and oxalosis, among others [1].

8. Conclusion

Atherosclerosis, arteriosclerosis and arteriolosclerosis are not only confused; they are also associated with some controversies. However, while the current classifications and description of terms have been developed over the centuries, there are possible better ways to classify the terms.

Author details

Oladimeji Adebayo[1*] and Abiodun Moshood Adeoye[1,2,3]

1 Cardiology Unit, Department of Medicine, University College Hospital, Ibadan, Nigeria

2 Department of Medicine, University of Ibadan, Ibadan, Nigeria

3 Cardiovascular Genetics and Genomic Research Unit, Institute of Cardiovascular Diseases, Faculty of Clinical Sciences, College of Medicine, University of Ibadan, Ibadan, Nigeria

*Address all correspondence to: doctorladi@gmail.com

IntechOpen

References

[1] Fishbein MC, Fishbein GA. Arteriosclerosis: Facts and fancy. Cardiovascular Pathology. 2015;24(6):335-342

[2] Fishbein GA, Fishbein MC. Arteriosclerosis: Rethinking the current classification. Archives of Pathology & Laboratory Medicine. 2009;133(8):1309-1316

[3] Schwartz C, Mitchell J. The morphology, terminology and pathogenesis of arterial plaques. Postgraduate Medical Journal. 1962;38(435):25

[4] McCullough PA et al. Accelerated atherosclerotic calcification and Mönckeberg's sclerosis: A continuum of advanced vascular pathology in chronic kidney disease. Clinical Journal of the American Society of Nephrology. 2008;3(6):1585-1598

[5] Schaar JA et al. Terminology for high-risk and vulnerable coronary artery plaques. European Heart Journal. 2004;25(12):1077-1082

[6] Lotufo PA. New findings about atherosclerosis in Brazil from the Brazilian Longitudinal Study of Adult Health (ELSA-Brasil). Sao Paulo Medical Journal. 2016;134(3):185-186

[7] Pickering SG. Arteriosclerosis and atherosclerosis: The need for clear thinking. The American Journal of Medicine. 1963;34(1):7-18

[8] Thomas GS et al. Why did ancient people have atherosclerosis?: From autopsies to computed tomography to potential causes. Global Heart. 2014;9(2):229-237

[9] Rabson SM. Arteriosclerosis: Definitions. American Journal of Clinical Pathology. 1954;24(4):472-473

[10] Hueper WJ. Arteriosclerosis. Archives of Pathology. 1945;39:187-216

[11] Stary HC et al. A definition of advanced types of atherosclerotic lesions and a histological classification of atherosclerosis. Circulation. 1995;92:1355-1374

[12] Sakata N. AGEs and atherosclerosis. Anti-Aging Medicine. 2012;9(3):89-95. Department of Pathology, Faculty of Medicine, Fukuoka University

[13] Fishbein GA, Fishbein MC. Arteriosclerosis. Archives of Pathology & Laboratory Medicine. 2009;133(8)

[14] Wilkinson IB, McEniery CM, Cockcroft JR. Arteriosclerosis and atherosclerosis: Guilty by association. American Heart Association. 2009;54:1213-1215

[15] Soltero-Perez I. Toward a new definition of atherosclerosis including hypertension: A proposal. Journal of Human Hypertension. 2002;16(S1):S23

[16] Hansson GK. Inflammation, atherosclerosis, and coronary artery disease. New England Journal of Medicine. 2005;352(16):1685-1695

[17] Ross R. Atherosclerosis—An inflammatory disease. New England Journal of Medicine. 1999;340(2):115-126

[18] Rafieian-Kopaei M et al. Atherosclerosis: Process, indicators, risk factors and new hopes. International Journal of Preventive Medicine. 2014;5(8):927-946

[19] Bridges LR et al. Blood-brain barrier dysfunction and cerebral small vessel disease (arteriolosclerosis) in brains of older people. Journal of Neuropathology

& Experimental Neurology. 2014;**73**(11):1026-1033

[20] Kryscio RJ et al. The effect of vascular neuropathology on late-life cognition: Results from the SMART project. The Journal of Prevention of Alzheimer's Disease. 2016;**3**(2):85-91

[21] Ighodaro ET et al. Risk factors and global cognitive status related to brain arteriolosclerosis in elderly individuals. Journal of Cerebral Blood Flow Metabolism. 2017;**37**(1):201-216

[22] Amann K. Media calcification and intima calcification are distinct entities in chronic kidney disease. Clinical Journal of the American Society of Nephrology. 2008;**3**(6):1599-1605

[23] Saxena A et al. Monckeberg medial calcific sclerosis mimicking malignant calcification pattern at mammography. Journal of Clinical Pathology. 2005;**58**(4):447-448

[24] Micheletti RG et al. Mönckeberg sclerosis revisited: A clarification of the histologic definition of Mönckeberg sclerosis. Archives of Pathology & Laboratory Medicine. 2008;**132**(1):43-47

[25] Hanke H, Lenz C, Finking G. The discovery of the pathophysiological aspects of atherosclerosis—A review. Acta Chirurgica Belgica. 2001;**101**(4):162-169

[26] Widmer L, Da Silva A. Historical perspectives and the Basle study. In: Epidemiology of Peripheral Vascular Disease. Springer; 1991. pp. 69-83

[27] Steinberg D. Thematic review series: the pathogenesis of atherosclerosis. An interpretive history of the cholesterol controversy: Part I. Journal of Lipid Research. 2004;**45**(9):1583-1593

[28] Hart GD et al. Lessons learned from the autopsy of an Egyptian mummy. Canadian Medical Association Journal. 1977;**117**(5):415

[29] Li J-J, Fang C-H. Atheroscleritis is a more rational term for the pathological entity currently known as atherosclerosis. Medical Hypotheses. 2004;**63**(1):100-102

[30] Cottet J, Lenoir M. Two thousand years of historical study on the words atheroma, atheromatosis, atherosclerosis, arteriosclerosis. Bulletin de l'Académie Nationale de Médecine. 1992;**176**(9):1385-1390. discussion 1390-1

[31] Widmer LK, Da Silva A. Historical perspectives and the basle study. In: Fowkes FGR, editor. Epidemiology of Peripheral Vascular Disease. London: Springer London; 1991. pp. 69-83

[32] Gaudio E et al. Morphological aspects of atherosclerosis lesion: Past and present. La Clinica Terapeutica. 2006;**157**(2):135-142

[33] Konstantinov IE, Mejevoi N, Anichkov NM, Nikolai N, et al. Anichkov and his theory of atherosclerosis. Texas Heart Institute Journal. 2006;**33**(4):417

[34] Ignatowski A. Über die Wirkung des tierischen Eiweisses auf die Aorta und die parenchymatösen Organe der Kaninchen. Virchows Archiv für Pathologische Anatomie und Physiologie und für Klinische Medizin. 1909;**198**(2):248-270

[35] Enas EA, Kuruvila AT, Lulla S. Retracing the heroic steps fromlipid hypothesis to aggressive treatment of blood cholesterol—A revolution in preventive cardiology. In: Choptra HK, Nanda Navin C, editors. Textbook of Cardiology. New Delhi: Jaypee Brothers Medical Publishers(P) Ltd; 2013. pp. 180-194

[36] Steinberg D. Thematic review series: The pathogenesis of atherosclerosis. An interpretive history of the cholesterol controversy, part V: the discovery of the statins and the end of the

controversy. Journal of Lipid Research. 2006;**47**(7):1339-1351

[37] Blumenthal HT. Cowdry's Arteriosclerosis: A Survey of the Problem. Thomas; 1967

[38] Drüeke TB. Arterial intima and media calcification: Distinct entities with different pathogenesis or all the same? Clinical Journal of the American Society of Nephrology. 2008;**3**(6):1583-1584

[39] André É, Lobstein J-F. Artériosclérose et ostéoporose. Société Française D'histoire De La Médecine. 2018;**52**:197

[40] Mönckeberg JG. Über die reine Mediaverkalkung der Extremitätenarterien und ihr Verhalten zur Arteriosklerose. Virchows Archiv für pathologische Anatomie und Physiologie und für klinische Medizin. 1903;**171**:141-167

[41] Marchand F. Ueber Atherosclerosis. Verhandlungen der Kongresse fuer Innere Medizin. 1904;**21**

[42] Windaus A. Über den Gehalt normaler und atheromatöser Aorten an Cholesterin und Cholesterinestern. Hoppe-Seyler's Zeitschrift für physiologische. Chemie. 1910;**67**(2): 174-176

[43] Anitschkow N. On experimental cholesterin steatosis and its significance in the origin of some pathological processes (1913). Arteriosclerosis. 1983;**3**:178-182

[44] Ross R, Klebanoff SJ. The smooth muscle cell: I. In vivo synthesis of connective tissue proteins. The Journal of Cell Biology. 1971;**50**(1):159-171

[45] Kondo T, Watanabe Y. A heritable hyperlipidemic rabbit. Jikken Dobutsu. 1975;**24**(3):89-94

Chapter 6

Coronary Atherosclerosis in Women

Abhishek Ojha and Nishtha Sareen

Abstract

Despite numerous studies focused on women's cardiac health, deaths from cardiovascular disease continue to rise in women. Cardiovascular disease (CVD) continues to be the leading cause of death even in women in many areas of the world. It has been noted that despite higher frequency of chest pain/angina in women compared to men, the incidence of obstructive coronary artery disease (CAD) remains lower in the female population compared with men presenting with similar symptoms. It is critical to have a deep understanding of these topics to ensure a meaningful communication between public, patients, and healthcare professionals. One reason to which this discrepancy has been attributed to is that chest pain in women is less likely to be secondary to obstructive coronary stenosis in comparison to men presenting with similar symptoms. The other issue is that the gold standard for coronary atherosclerosis continues to coronary angiography. This is a key limitation in cardiovascular atherosclerosis management since endothelial dysfunction in addition to a higher risk of atherosclerosis is prevalent in women with hypertension, diabetes, and dyslipidemia. In this chapter, we will focus on the aspects of coronary atherosclerosis that deserve attention with respect to gender-specific considerations, particularly with respect to clinical practice.

Keywords: atherosclerosis, coronary, myocardial infarction, females, gender

1. Introduction

Despite numerous studies focused on women's cardiac health, deaths from cardiovascular disease continue to rise in women. Cardiovascular disease (CVD) continues to be the leading cause of death even in women in many areas of the world. It has been note that despite higher frequency of chest pain/angina in women compared to men, the incidence of obstructive coronary artery disease (CAD) remains lower in the female population compared with men presenting with similar symptoms [1]. It is critical to have a deep understanding of these topics to ensure a meaningful communication between public, patients, and healthcare professionals.

It is important to note that despite all the literature diagnoses, cardiovascular illness in women remains underdeveloped. One of the reasons which it has been attributed to is that chest pain in women is less likely to be secondary to obstructive or flow-limiting coronary stenosis in comparison to men presenting with similar symptoms [1]. The other issue is that the gold standard for coronary atherosclerosis continues to coronary angiography [1]. This is a key limitation in cardiovascular atherosclerosis management since endothelial dysfunction, in addition to a higher risk of atherosclerosis is prevalent in women with hypertension, diabetes, and dyslipidemia [2].

Gianturco et al. [3] have also explained the role of systemic inflammation as a potential under-recognized player in endothelial dysfunction. Both inflammation and immunity seem to be the critical players [3]. The authors have emphasized on the need for preventive strategies after detailed understanding of the possible underlying pathogenesis [3].

In this chapter, we will focus on the aspects of coronary atherosclerosis that deserve attention with respect to gender specific considerations, particularly with respect to clinical practice.

2. Pathogenesis

Endothelial dysfunction, inflammation, and atheromatous plaque in women, as well as men, is primarily caused as a result of aging, dyslipidemia, hypertension, cigarette smoking, and diabetes. These five risk factors mentioned are all well-known traditional risk factors with well-documented correlation to pathophysiology of CAD [4].

2.1 Oral contraceptives and heart disease

Oral contraceptives (OC) have been associated with a higher risk of athero-sclerosis and venous thrombosis since their introduction in clinical practice [5]. The risk for acute heart attack was increased by a factor of 2.5 in those who used second-generation contraceptives when compared to third-generation OC (OR1.3) on comparison of the different generations of these medications. This suggests a lower risk in newer generation OC but the overall findings remain inconclusive. The authors, hence, concluded that the recommendation to health care providers should include a dedicated screen for traditional cardiovascular risk factors and events before prescribing OC [6].

2.2 Pregnancy and heart disease

Pregnancy is associated with elevated atherogenic responses, including insulin resistance and dyslipidemia, with consequent manifestation as preeclampsia and gestational diabetes. These complications can contribute to higher postpartum risk of CVD, with a two-fold increase in CAD and cerebrovascular disease [7]. Preeclampsia has been associated with insulin resistance, hypertension, lower high-density lipoprotein concentrations, higher plasma levels of triglycerides, high uric acid, and high levels of insulin. This is in addition to its recognition as a state of sympathetic overactivity and proinflammatory changes [7]. Thus, preeclampsia should be carefully evaluated as a potential index manifestation of the metabolic syndrome.

2.3 Parity and heart disease

There is a well-established relationship between number of children, CAD risk factors and prevalent CAD in both women and men in the age range of 60–79 years [8].

The comparison of gender indexes helps delineate whether the association is secondary to biological processes or due to lifestyle factors. The results have consistently shown an association of increasing number of children with increasing obesity in both sexes. In women alone, there was suggestion of association between number of children and CAD, even after adjustment for obesity and metabolic factors [8].

2.4 ACS in women

A detailed review of the Rapid Early Action for Coronary Treatment (REACT) study designed by the NHLBI was performed, which tested multistrategy campaigns to reduce patient delay to seek care for ACS symptoms [9]. It was clearly shown that reducing the time to treatment was associated with significantly lower rates of death and disability caused by AMI [9]. This is critical information for education not only of the healthcare providers, but also of patients, individual women and the general public. Timely recognition of symptoms of ACS with prompt medical response to early symptoms can be lifesaving.

The study has, hence, made some direct recommendations. One is patient awareness of symptoms in addition to chest pain, pressure, or discomfort. In addition, the fact is that the symptoms may not be dramatic or sudden. The recognition of symptoms by women in the community and the healthcare providers in female patients requires further research. This research should focus on the prodromal syndromes with dedicated dissemination of public messages and information aimed at healthcare providers. Lastly, the NHLBI document diligently encourages better understanding of all pathophysiological basis of ACS in women with the intention to optimize treatment recommendations.

2.5 Endothelial dysfunction

Endothelium interacts with nearly each and every system of the human body, with definite implication in end organ diseases of systems including neurologic, renal, hepatic, vascular, dermatologic, immunologic, and cardiac [10]. Additionally, the endothelium regulates vascular tone, maintaining careful balance between vasoconstriction and vasodilation with the intention to provide adequate perfusion pressure to target organs. Additional functions include regulation of angiogenesis, wound healing, smooth muscle cell proliferation, fibrosis, and inflammation [10]. Interestingly, the factors that adversely affect the endothelium are also the common cardiovascular risk factors such as tobacco use, obesity, age, hypertension, hyperlipidemia, physical inactivity, and poor dietary habits [10].

3. Management strategies of atherosclerosis in women

It has been shown in studies that in female patients with coronary artery disease, persistent impairment of endothelial vasomotor function despite optimized therapy to reduce risk factors can adversely affect clinical outcomes [11].

The following, however, should be aggressively managed to combat atherosclerotic disease in female patients:

1. Life style modifications (diet, exercise, smoking, weight reduction)

Adherence with healthy eating habits, regular exercising and weight reduction are all important determinants of atherosclerosis and should be recommended in both genders [12]. Smoking cessation is critical and dedicated time should be spent with patients to generate that awareness [12].

2. Receptor and enzyme pathways (beta-blockers, ET, ACE-I, ARB)

Just as the traditional risk factors play a critical role in the pathogenesis of atherosclerotic CAD in females, the routine therapies should be considered in this patient population [13].

Most studies have found the benefit of statins in ameliorating and even eliminating endothelial dysfunction [13]. These medications are well known mainstay in decreasing CVD risk in most patients secondary to their lipid-lowering and anti-inflammatory mechanism [13]. Addition of ACE-inhibition to statin therapy has been shown to improve endothelial-dependent relaxation in the coronary vasculature through NO-dependent mechanism [14, 15].

3. NO pathway (L-arginine, PDE-I)

Both intravenous and intracoronary administration of L-arginine, the physiologic precursor for NO, has been shown to acutely improve endothelium-dependent, but not endothelium-independent, vasodilation in participants with hypercholesterolemia or CAD [16]. The longer-term effects of oral L-arginine have additionally been evaluated. Among patients who have underlying heart failure, oral L-arginine improved endothelial function, arterial compliance, and functional status [17].

The other agent is Nicorandil, which is a potent antianginal, however, unavailable in the US. It has dual nitrate and potassium-ATP channel agonist properties and increases the formation of cyclic GMP. This agent has been shown to improve endothelial function in patients without prior CAD at 1 year follow up with concomitant documented reductions in inflammatory markers [18].

4. Channel pathways (Ca, K)

Nifedipine has been shown to have antioxidant effects with additional effect on endothelial nitric oxide synthase expression. In a study including 454 patients undergoing percutaneous coronary intervention, endothelium dependent vasodilatation was evaluated with intracoronary acetylcholine following 6 months of therapy with nifedipine. There was well documented improvement in endothelial function, however, no plaque regression [19].

Ranolazine is a sodium channel inhibitor used in patients who have refractory angina. It has been shown to improve symptoms of microvascular angina, however there was no clear change seen in microvascular function with the use of ranolazine [20].

4. Conclusion

In summary, atherosclerosis in females is a complex process. There is an integral role of endothelial dysfunction. In order to close the gaps in care of cardiac disease in women, the steps must include timely recognition of the symptoms of cardiac disease with the effective management. Treatment strategies are diverse with decent evidence base. Larger studies dedicated to address atherosclerosis in women are urgently required.

Author details

Abhishek Ojha[1*] and Nishtha Sareen[2]

1 Independent Scientist, Michigan, United States

2 Ascension Providence Hospital, Michigan, United States

*Address all correspondence to: dr.abhishekojha@gmail.com

IntechOpen

References

[1] Kennedy JW, Killip T, Fisher LD, et al. The clinical spectrum of coronary artery disease and its surgical and medical management, 1974-1979. The coronary artery surgery study. Circulation. 1982;**66**:III-16-III-23

[2] Quyyumi AA. Endothelial function in health and disease: New insights into the genesis of cardiovascular disease. The American Journal of Medicine. 1998;**105**:32S-39S

[3] Giarturco L, Bodini BD, Atzeni F, Colombo C, Stella D, Sarzi-Puttini P, et al. Cardiovascular and autoimmune diseases in females: The role of microvasculature and dysfunctional endothelium. Atherosclerosis. 2014;**241**(1):259-263

[4] Sharret AR, Ballantyne CM, Coady SA, et al. Coronary heart disease prediction from lipoprotein cholesterol levels, triglycerides, lipoprotein(a), apolipoproteins A-I and B, and HDL density subfractions: The Atherosclerosis Risk in Communities (ARIC) study. Circulation. 2001;**104**:1108-1113

[5] Tanis BC, Rosendaal FR. Venous and arterial thrombosis during oral contraceptive use: Risks and risk factors. Seminars in Vascular Medicine. 2003;**3**:69-84

[6] Tanis BC, Van den Bosch MAAJ, Kemmeren JM, et al. Oral contraceptives and the risk of myocardial infarction. The New England Journal of Medicine. 2001;**345**:1787-1793

[7] Kaaja RJ, Greer IA. Manifestations of chronic disease during pregnancy. Journal of the American Medical Association. 2005;**294**:2751-2757

[8] Lawlor DA, Emberson JR, Ebrahim S, et al. Is the association between parity and coronary heart disease due to biological effects of pregnancy or adverse lifestyle risk factors associated with child-rearing? Circulation. 2003;**107**:1260-1264

[9] Simons-Morton DG, Goff DC, Osganian S, et al. Rapid early action for coronary treatment: Rationale, design and baseline characteristics. Academic Emergency Medicine: Official Journal of the Society for Academic Emergency Medicine. 1998;**5**:726-738

[10] Araujo LF, de Matos Soeiro A, Fernandes JL, Pesaro AE, Serrano CV Jr. Coronary artery disease in women: A review on prevention, pathophysiology, diagnosis, and treatment. Vascular Health and Risk Management. 2006;**2**(4):465-475. DOI: 10.2147/vhrm.2006.2.4.465

[11] Kitta Y, Obata JE, Nakamura T, Hirano M, Kodama Y, Fujioka D, et al. Persistent impairment of endothelial vasomotor function has a negative impact on outcome in patients with coronary artery disease. Journal of the American College of Cardiology. 2009;**53**(4):323-330

[12] Prasad A, Tupas-Habib T, Schenke WH, Mincemoyer R, Panza JA, Waclawin MA, et al. Quyyumi acute and chronic angiotensin-1 receptor antagonism reverses endothelial dysfunction in atherosclerosis. Circulation. 2000;**101**(20):2349-2354

[13] Bonetti PO, Lerman LO, Lerman A. Endothelial dysfunction: A marker of atherosclerotic risk. Arteriosclerosis, Thrombosis, and Vascular Biology. 2003;**23**(2):168-175

[14] Hinoi T, Tomohiro Y, Kajiwara S, Matsuo S, Fujimoto Y, Yamamoto S, et al. Telmisartan, an angiotensin II type 1 receptor blocker, improves

coronary microcirculation and insulin resistance among essential hypertensive patients without left ventricular hypertrophy. Hypertension Research. 2008;**31**(4):615-622

[15] Tiefenbacher CP, Friedrich S, Bleeke T, Vahl C, Chen X, Niroomand F. et al. ACE inhibitors and statins acutely improve endothelial dysfunction of human coronary arterioles. American Journal of Physiology. Heart and Circulatory Physiology. 2004;**286**(4):H1425-H1432

[16] Bonetti PO, Pumper GM, Higano ST, Holmes DR Jr, Kuvin JT, Lerman A. Noninvasive identification of patients with early coronary atherosclerosis by assessment of digital reactive hyperemia. Journal of the American College of Cardiology. 2004;**44**(11):2137-2141

[17] Modena MG, Bonetti L, Coppi F, Bursi F, Rossi R. Prognostic role of reversible endothelial dysfunction in hypertensive postmenopausal women. Journal of the American College of Cardiology. 2002;**40**(3):505-510

[18] Ishibashi Y, Takahashi N, Tokumaru A, Karino K, Sugamori T, Sakane T, et al. Effects of long-term nicorandil administration on endothelial function, inflammation, and oxidative stress in patients without coronary artery disease. Journal of Cardiovascular Pharmacology. 2008;**51**(3):311-316

[19] Lüscher TF, Pieper M, Tendera M, Vrolix M, Rutsch W, van den Branden F, et al. A randomized placebo-controlled study on the effect of nifedipine on coronary endothelial function and plaque formation in patients with coronary artery disease: The ENCORE II study. European Heart Journal. 2009;**30**(13):1590-1597

[20] Villano A, Di Franco A, Nerla R, Sestito A, Tarzia P, Lamendola P, et al.

Effects of ivabradine and ranolazine in patients with microvascular angina pectoris. The American Journal of Cardiology. 2013;**112**(1):8-13